D0079627

# HEALTH AND WELLNESS
## IN ANTIQUITY THROUGH THE MIDDLE AGES

# HEALTH AND WELLNESS
## IN ANTIQUITY THROUGH THE MIDDLE AGES

WILLIAM H. YORK

Health and Wellness in Daily Life
*Joseph P. Byrne, Series Editor*

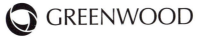 GREENWOOD

AN IMPRINT OF ABC-CLIO, LLC
Santa Barbara, California • Denver, Colorado • Oxford, England

**Library of Congress Cataloging-in-Publication Data**

York, William Henry, 1968–
    Health and wellness in antiquity through the Middle Ages / William H. York.
        p. ; cm. — (Health and wellness in daily life)
    Includes bibliographical references and index.
    ISBN 978-0-313-37865-2 (hardcopy : alk. paper) —
    ISBN 978-0-313-37866-9 (ebook)
I. Title.   II. Series: Health and wellness in daily life.
[DNLM:  1. Health—history.   2. History of Medicine.
3. History, Ancient.   4. History, Medieval.   WZ 51]
    610.938—dc23        2012011917

ISBN: 978-0-313-37865-2
EISBN: 978-0-313-37866-9

16   15   14   13   12      1   2   3   4   5

This book is also available on the World Wide Web as an eBook.
Visit www.abc-clio.com for details.

Greenwood
An Imprint of ABC-CLIO, LLC

ABC-CLIO, LLC
130 Cremona Drive, P.O. Box 1911
Santa Barbara, California 93116-1911

This book is printed on acid-free paper ∞

Manufactured in the United States of America

For my boys,
Arthur and Galen,
and most especially my wife,
Michelle,
with love.

# Contents

# Series Foreword

Communities have few concerns that are as fundamental as the health of their members. America's current concern for societal provision of health care is as much a political, ethical, economic, and social matter as it is a technical or "medical" one. Reflection on the history of health and medicine may help us to place our contemporary concerns in context, but it also shows how far humanity has come in being able and willing to provide for the highest levels of health and health care possible. It is a reminder, too, of the possibilities the future presents. Our culture believes in progress, but it is also aware that unforeseen challenges will continue to appear. Health and medicine are cultural as well as biological constructs, and we live each day with the constraints and opportunities that follow.

This series of seven monographs explores the courses that human health and medicine have taken from antiquity to the present day. Though far from being complete in their coverage, these volumes map out continuities and changes over time in a set of health and medical fields. Each author has taken on the same outline in order to allow the student of health, medicine, and history to discover conditions, beliefs, practices, and changes within a given period, but also to trace the same concerns across time and place. With this in mind, each volume contains chapters on, for example, healers, children's health and healing, occupational and environmental threats, and epidemic disease. To the extent possible, we authors have attempted to emphasize the ways in which these have affected people in their daily lives, rather than viewing them through the lenses of the healers or their profession. Our hope is that these volumes constitute a small and very useful library of the history of health and medicine.

As editor, I have endeavored to bring on board authors who are medical historians as well as fine teachers who have the ability to transmit their knowledge in writing with the same enthusiasm they bring into the classroom. As an author, I am sharing the discoveries, the joys, and not least the challenges and frustrations that all of us encounter in producing this series.

*Joseph P. Byrne*
Honors Program
Belmont University

# CHAPTER 1

# Factors in Health and Wellness

## HEALTH AND DISEASE IN HISTORY

In early hunter and gatherer societies, with small, scattered populations, humans were unlikely to have been exposed to numerous contagious bacterial and viral diseases that require large, dense populations to spread (such as smallpox). Furthermore, the nomadic lifestyle of these early societies would have minimized the possibility of contact with water polluted by human waste and piles of refuse and garbage that might attract disease-carrying insects. Finally, prior to the period of widespread domestication of animals, these peoples were less likely to contract diseases passed on by close contact with dogs, pigs, birds, and cattle, not to mention the mice and rats drawn to human dwellings. This is not to say that early humans lived without disease; indeed they still faced a number of diseases caused by eating animals, or passed on by worms and lice. The limited population sizes, however, would have limited incidences of infection and death from infectious diseases. As humans began to live together in larger, permanent settlements starting around 10,000 B.C.E., they encountered a whole new range of diseases of civilization. Living in cities brought humans into closer, regular contact with pathogens and parasites that were spread by contact with domesticated animals, or through poor sanitation and fouled water supplies. The larger and denser populations also made it easier for infectious diseases to spread, allowing some (like smallpox and measles) that had previously caused little trouble to emerge and thrive. Furthermore, archaeological evidence indicates that as humans started to live in permanent settlements and rely on agriculture and domesticated animals for food, their diets became less varied and focused on a limited number of staple crops, leading to malnutrition from not getting appropriate nutrients. The changed diets would only further enable the spread of diseases due to weakened immunities. Clearly, the move to civilization brought a trade-off—on the one hand it may have allowed for increased security, but on the other, it led to an increase in disease. In this context, the need for effective means of treating disease became even more crucial once humans started to congregate in cities.

Faced with these conditions, humans in the earliest civilizations began to develop theories about health and disease and to recognize different professionals in society who were deemed proficient in the craft of healing. This book is about the early medical beliefs and practices in civilizations from around the world from their earliest origins in antiquity until roughly 1500 C.E. We will focus on the medical traditions in seven different premodern societies: Mesopotamia (ca. 3000–500 B.C.E.), Egypt (ca. 3000–300 B.C.E.), Greece and Rome (ca. 1200 B.C.E.–500 C.E.), India (ca. 2000 B.C.E.–1400 C.E.), China (ca. 2000 B.C.E.–1400 C.E.), the Islamic World (ca. seventh century–1400 C.E.), and the European Middle Ages (ca. 500–1450 C.E.). The broad geographic scope will allow us to recognize the distinct beliefs and practices and how they developed in relation to the cultural beliefs of each individual civilization. At the same time, however, when viewed together they display the commonality of approaches human societies have taken toward a shared interest in preserving health and curing disease.

Some of the explanations for disease, theories about the body, methods of treatment, and kinds of practitioners we will consider in this book may bear little relation to the medical beliefs and practices with which we ourselves are familiar in the twenty-first century. Indeed, one might feel tempted by the strangeness of some of the medical systems to dismiss them as superstitious, irrational, and even dangerous. Or, we might choose to recognize only those beliefs and practices that appear to suggest the origins of our own modern, scientific medical ideas. In following either of those temptations, however, we would fail to recognize the complexities of medical decisions faced by our predecessors in the earliest human civilizations and the innovative means by which they sought to address them. Furthermore, although some of the medical traditions examined in this book have fallen into disuse, others (the Indian and Chinese medical traditions) are still regularly practiced and continue to develop around the world today. Increasingly in the West, many people are turning to so-called alternative medical beliefs, which are often based on the ancient traditions we will examine here. We must, therefore, recognize that the medical theories and procedures valued in any given society are determined as much by cultural beliefs as by any objective measure of the efficacy of the treatments. As such, the ability to view these medical traditions together should remind us that healing is a social activity, and the decisions a society makes about how to treat the sick, injured, and disabled are reflective of its most sacred beliefs and cultural values.

## HEALTH, DISEASE, AND THE BODY

In the Hippocratic text *Epidemics I*, the author states that "the art [of medicine] has three factors: the disease, the patient, the physician. The physician is the servant of the art. The patient must cooperate with the physician in combating the disease" (Jones 1984, 165). We will consider the roles of physicians and patients in later chapters, but we should examine definitions of disease and health here. Indeed, explanations for what constitutes disease vary over time and cultural context, as do the meanings associated with being diagnosed with having a particular condition. In many cases, the definitions are closely linked with conceptions about the functioning of the body, and hence it is necessary to consider theories about the body's anatomy and physiology when seeking to understand beliefs about the causes and processes of disease. Therefore, before we examine the development of the different healing practices and the health care practitioners associated with each, it will be useful first to examine the theoretical explanations for what constitutes disease and how it works in the body according to the different medical traditions.

### Disease Theory in the Ancient Near East: Mesopotamia and Egypt

Mesopotamian healers had little theoretical knowledge of anatomy or physiology. They identified the heart as the site of intelligence, the liver as the source of anger, and the kidneys as the foundation of strength. Furthermore, they also recognized that various parts of the body (e.g., the chest or the guts) could become inflamed, but there was no systematic explanation for the disease process in the body. Rather, the Mesopotamian medical tradition held that disease was caused by gods, demons, evil spirits, or magic. Accordingly, treatment in the

Mesopotamian tradition was mostly directed toward combating those external causes of sickness through appropriate rituals, incantations, and sacrifices. The demonic or magical explanation for the cause of disease could imply that the sick person was in some way at fault for the illness, receiving the curse as a punishment for some offense they had committed. Belief in the religious and magical causes of disease also necessitated that those responsible for treating disease should be the priests and magicians who could perform the necessary rituals to exorcise the offending spirit from the body. Likewise, the preservation of health required that the individual seek to maintain an appropriate state of spiritual purity by following the appropriate practices to pacify the demons or supernatural beings, who might cause disease. We shall look more closely at the role of religious and magical healing in Mesopotamian society in a later chapter. For now, it suffices to note that the Mesopotamian belief system did not require a detailed understanding of the body or the causes of disease within the body.

In the Egyptian tradition, we find a blend of religious/magical explanations with naturalistic explanations for disease. The naturalistic understanding of disease causation explained how disease worked within the body as a natural (not magical) process. Egyptian physicians believed that the body was filled with a network of vessels or channels, called *metu*, which included blood vessels, ducts, tendons, and muscles. The *metu* were believed to originate in the heart from which they extended to different parts of the body, so that the heart could "speak" through them. The various *metu* were believed ultimately to unite again at the anus, thus making them ideal channels by which a variety of substances—including blood, air, mucus, urine, semen, feces, various disease-bearing entities, and good or evil spirits—could be transported through the body. The large number of remedies aimed at strengthening or softening the *metu*, which could become mute or even die, indicate just how important these vessels were to the Egyptian understanding of the body and disease.

In addition to carrying useful materials through the body, the *metu* were believed to be the channels through which *wekhedu* traveled. Although scholars continue to debate the meaning of the term *wekhedu* (suggestions include "pain" or "purulency"), the best translation is likely "morbid (disease-causing) principle." In theory, *wekhedu* originated in the anus (although it was distinct from feces) and spread through the *metu* to the rest of the body, where it caused abscesses, pain, and a variety of different kinds of diseases. Based on the recognition of the fact that the bowels were the first part of the body to putrefy after death, Egyptian theorists believed that the bowels were the source of putrefaction and hence *wekhedu* in the body. Thus, many remedies were designed for the care of the anus, to help expel *wekhedu* by means of regular medicinal purges and enemas.

## Disease Theory in the Western Medical Tradition: Greece, Rome, the Islamic World, and Medieval Europe

The earliest Greek medical writings are the books of the Hippocratic Corpus, the roughly sixty texts written between about 420 and 350 B.C.E. and ascribed to Hippocrates of Cos, a doctor famed for teaching medicine in the fifth century B.C.E. The authors of these books sought to provide a naturalistic explanation for health and disease in terms of the physiological functioning of the body. The Hippocratic theories, which originated in the fifth and fourth centuries B.C.E. and were subsequently modified and clarified by later Greek authors, most importantly Aristotle (384–322 B.C.E.) and Galen (129–ca. 216 C.E.), provided the essential philosophy for understanding the mechanisms of disease in Western Europe into the eighteenth century. Furthermore, the Hippocratic theories were also adopted by early Arabic medical authors and hence provided the foundation for Islamic medical theory as well. Arabic and European physicians continued to refine and augment the theoretical model they inherited from the Greeks over the course of more than 1,000 years. In this section we shall examine the core elements of this system, which came to be referred to as humoralism.

In their efforts to understand and explain the natural order of the cosmos without attributing natural events to the actions of gods, Greek pre-Socratic philosophers sought to identify the primary constituents out of which the universe was composed. Numerous competing answers existed for this question, and it was not until a much later period that the theoretical model proposed by Empedocles (ca. 490–430 B.C.E.) became predominant. According to Empedocles, all matter in the universe was believed to be composed of a specific combination of the four basic elementary substances (fire, air, water, and earth). The elemental theory sought to explain the process of change in the universe in terms of the strife between opposed pairs of elements (air-earth, fire-water) and the attraction between other elements (e.g., air has properties in common with fire and water).

In the same period, authors of the Hippocratic medical texts considered the essential building blocks of the body, and they too proposed a number of competing answers. Various Hippocratic texts suggest that the body included one or more essential fluids called *chymoi*, which is usually translated as "humors." In the second century C.E., the famous Greek physician Galen of Pergamum emphasized the theory proposed

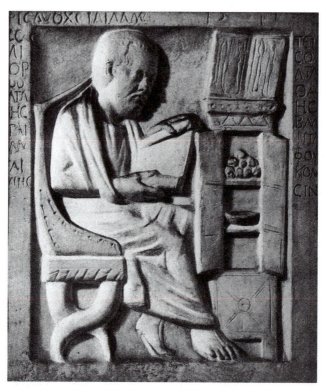

This bas-relief from a Roman sarcophagus from about 100 C.E. shows a doctor reading a scroll before a cabinet, which contains other scrolls and a bowl, likely used for collecting blood when bloodletting. The doctor's surgical instruments rest on top of the cabinet. The image emphasizes both the doctor's theoretical learning from books and his practical skills in surgery. (Hulton Archive/Getty Images)

in the Hippocratic text *On the Nature of Man* that the body contained four humors: blood, phlegm, bile (often called yellow bile or choler), and black bile (or melancholy). Blood, bile, and phlegm were observed being excreted in times of illness or injury and correlate to fluids we recognize today. Modern scholars continue to debate what bodily fluid black bile might be associated with, but it was supposed to be visible in vomit and excreta. These humors were believed to combine in the body to regulate its proper functioning; even the blood found in the veins was considered to consist of a mixture of humoral blood with the three other humors, so that one might be able to separate out the other humors from venous blood.

Galen also credited Hippocrates with the concept of the four opposing qualities (hot, cold, wet, and dry), although this concept is normally attributed to Aristotle. Galen's efforts presented a unified system for drawing connections between the body (microcosm) and the greater universe (macrocosm). In this system, each of the humors was likened to one of the four elements, and furthermore, each element/humor was described as manifesting two of the basic qualities, so that, for example, blood was linked to the element air and both were described as being hot and wet, while phlegm was linked with the element water, and they were cold and wet (see Figure 1.1). The explanatory power of this scheme extended further to identify each humor with the four seasons, the four winds, the four ages of man (childhood, youth, adulthood, and old age) and later with different heavenly bodies and signs of the zodiac, and among Christian scholars, with the four Evangelists. In this way, the actions of the humors in the body could be understood in terms of macrocosmic influences whereby seasonal changes and other environmental conditions might cause an elevation in certain humors (e.g., blood became more prevalent in the spring) possibly leading to disease.

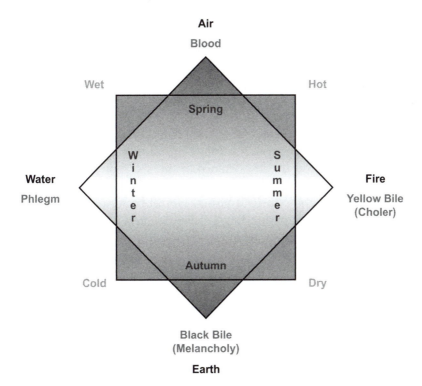

**Figure 1.1** The humoral system.

One of the most fundamental ideas in the Hippocratic Corpus is the notion that health requires balance, while disease results from imbalance in the body. According to the humoral theory, imbalance was normally conceived of as an excess of one or more humors, and it might be systemic (affecting the entire body) or localized (in a specific part of the body), depending on the disease. Fevers were viewed as diseases of the whole body, while diseases like catarrh (a respiratory infection accompanied by a cough) and podagra (gout, an infection in the feet) resulted from an excess of one humor in a specific area of the body (in the chest and feet, respectively). During the Middle Ages, each person was thought to have his or her own individual healthy balance of humors, referred to as one's temperament or complexion, in which it was possible for one of the humors to predominate. For example, a person whose healthy balance of humors contained a little more blood than the other humors would be referred to as being sanguine, one with a little more yellow bile was choleric, one with more phlegm was phlegmatic, and one in whom black bile dominated was melancholic. The different temperamental types might be more prone to different kinds of diseases and may require slightly modified forms treatment. The exact nature of the imbalance might be diagnosed by careful observation of a number of signs or symptoms, but following Galen, doctors specifically examined the pulse and the urine. Treatment of disease would aim at restoring balance in the body by purging excess humors (e.g., through bloodletting or inducing vomiting) or countering the excess with pharmaceutical remedies.

Numerous factors might influence an individual's humoral balance, and physicians emphasized that health could be restored through the careful adjustment of those factors. Beginning with Galen, medical scholars emphasized the importance of the six "non-naturals," environmental, physiological, and psychological conditions that affected health and over which the individual would have some control. The non-naturals are the surrounding air, exercise and rest, sleep and waking, food and drink, retention and excretion, and the "accidents of the soul." The environmental influence of the surrounding air would include exposure to any areas of stagnant, putrescent, or foul-smelling airs found near swamps, crypts, or other places with close proximity to decaying matter. The other non-naturals existed in a state of balance in which the individual would be expected to adjust his levels of activity (including coitus) and rest as well as diet and excretion. Likewise, the individual should control the "accidents of the soul," which included the passions and emotions, to maintain an appropriate mental balance. If these conditions were not sufficiently regulated, then shifts in the humoral balance would lead the body to succumb to a contra-natural (against nature), or diseased state. Thus, in his *Isagoge* (*Introduction to Medicine*), the Eastern Christian physician Hunayn ibn Ishaq (d. ca. 873 or 877), known as Johannitius in the West, wrote about the need to consider the effect of the foods people ate on their humors, noting that "foods are of two kinds: good food is that which brings about a good humor, and bad food is that which brings about an evil humor." For example, he indicated that fresh bread and lamb produce healthy blood, mustard and garlic beget yellow bile, cabbage and the meat of old goats make black bile, while pork produces phlegm (Cholmeley 1912, 145–146). Furthermore, seasonal shifts and weather changes might cause the body's humoral balance to shift in response, meaning that the individual would need to monitor her diet and regimen continually with regard to other environmental conditions. In addition to regulating diet and exercise, individuals could take other prophylactic measures in response to seasonal influences on the body; for example, people would be sure to receive a preventative bloodletting in the spring (the season when blood, the hot and wet humor, would rise) to guard against diseases caused by excess blood.

## Disease Theory in Indian Ayurvedic Medicine

From an early stage, Indian Ayurvedic medicine developed a highly complex theoretical understanding of the body and how it related to the origin and progress of disease. The central belief of Ayurvedic disease theory revolves around the concept of the three *doshas*, or humors, which are responsible for the proper functioning of the body: *vata* (wind or air), *pitta* (bile or fire), and *kapha* (phlegm or water). Although the *doshas* are found throughout the body, each one is believed to have a primary seat within a particular part of the body where it tends to congregate and have the greatest influence: *vata* (colon, large intestines), *pitta* (small intestines), *kapha* (lungs, chest). Learned Indian doctors, like Greek medical philosophers, believed in a correspondence between the human body (microcosm) and the universe (macrocosm) and regarded each of the *doshas* as being composed of two of the five constituent elements of the cosmos (ether, air, fire, water, earth). Thus, according to a system of correspondence, the body's internal *doshas* are linked to the macrocosm so that *vata* is believed to be composed of ether and air, *pitta* is composed of fire and water, and *kapha* is composed of water and earth. Furthermore, the balance in the body of the quantity and quality of the *doshas* can be affected by numerous macrocosmic and microcosmic factors, including the food eaten, the level of physical activity, the climate, and the age and emotional state of the individual.

In addition to the *doshas*, there are other components of the body that are regarded as significant in the disease process, especially the *dhatus*, the *ojas*, and the *malas*. The *dhatus*, the seven basic structural constituents (tissues and fluids) of the body, evolve in sequence from the most gross to the more compact and refined, with each forming and nourishing the following one in turn. *Rasa* (plasma or chyle), the largest material substance, produces *rakta* (blood), followed by *mamsa* (muscle and flesh), *meda* (fat), *asthi* (bone), *majjan* (marrow and nerve tissue), which forms the most refined of the *dhatus*, *shukra* (semen). In addition to the *dhatus*, another product of the process of nutrition and digestion is *ojas*, which is perhaps best identified as an essence of vitality or energy. *Ojas* can be depleted by anxiety, anger, depression, hunger, pain, and excessive physical exercise, leading to ill health. In addition to the fundamental elements of the *dhatus* and *ojas*, the body also produces three main waste products, *malas*, as a result of the process of digestion: feces, urine, and sweat. The maintenance of health requires that the *malas* be effectively eliminated from the body, but they also play an essential role in the body. For example, feces is important for helping to separate waste from nutritive materials, while sweat is believed to be valuable for regulating the body's temperature and moistening the skin. Disproportions of the *dhatus* and *malas* manifested various signs in the body. For example, the loss of lymph chyle would lead to pain about the region of the heart, heart palpitations, and thirst; loss of blood would be marked by a roughness of the skin, a craving for acidic foods or drinks, and "loose and flabby" veins; the loss or scanty formation of fecal matter would cause a sensation of pain in the sides and around the heart, accompanied by gas and a rumbling sound in the intestines and in the region of the liver.

In Ayurvedic medicine, the process through which the *dhatus* and *malas* are produced is regulated by the *agni* or fire. *Agni*, imbued with a transformative power, is a digestive force by which one substance absorbs and assimilates nutrients and is changed into another. Traditional Ayurvedic medical texts recognize several forms of *agni*, each responsible for different transformative actions, including processing the five elements in foods so that they can be absorbed by the body, directing the metabolic process for the creation of the *dhatus* and *malas*, and even, on the psychological level, assisting transformations in thought and feeling. The other essential components of the digestive process are the *srotas*, an interconnected network of channels or tubes in the body through which *doshas*, nutrients, and waste materials are transported to the *dhatus* and organs. Each system of *srotas* is associated with a different organ or part of the body, and hence a disruption in an organ would produce ill effects throughout its network of *srotas*.

Ayurveda recognizes health as a state of harmony when the *doshas* exist in the optimal quality and quantity in the appropriate areas, and when the *agni* and the *srotas* together maintain proper digestion and allow for the proper distribution of nutrients to the body for the production of *dhatus* and ensure the timely removal of *malas*. Most important, the maintenance of health requires that the *doshas* remain in a proper state of equilibrium, existing in the normal quantity in the appropriate parts of the body without becoming irritated or inflamed. However, diet, lifestyle, and psychological stress (in addition to age and seasonal changes) can all adversely affect the state of the *doshas* and thus compromise an individual's health. The disruption of the *doshas* can, in turn, impair the *agni* and the digestive process, which could lead to blockages in the *srotas* and compromise timely removal of *malas* and the proper functioning of the *dhatus* and other organs. Furthermore, when the *agni* is impaired the body is more prone to producing *ama*, a kind of toxic waste substance resulting from inefficient digestion that can cause disease. Finally, the proper level of *ojas* in the body also plays an important part in health, and when digestion is disrupted this level decreases, further weakening the body's vitality and ability to resist disease. An Ayurvedic physician, therefore, needs to consider a complex series of interlocking factors relating to the body when attempting to diagnose the cause of a patient's illness.

Ayurvedic medicine emphasizes the idea that health not only entails a physical condition but also requires mental and spiritual wholeness and integration. The proper preservation of health, therefore, necessitates that the individual not only maintain a harmonious balance of physiological functioning but also achieve a state of consciousness in which his or her emotional state and cognitive awareness are also in alignment with the body. This holistic view of health attends to far more than physical and mental conditions but also seeks to consider the spiritual and social interconnectedness of the individual. In this way, Ayurvedic medicine has several points of commonality with other practices like yoga, which encourages meditation and active poses aimed at bringing body, mind, and spirit into harmony with one another.

### Disease Theory in Traditional Chinese Medicine

The body in traditional Chinese medicine is conceived as interacting with the universe according to an intricate theory of systematic correspondences. This theoretical system originated during the Han

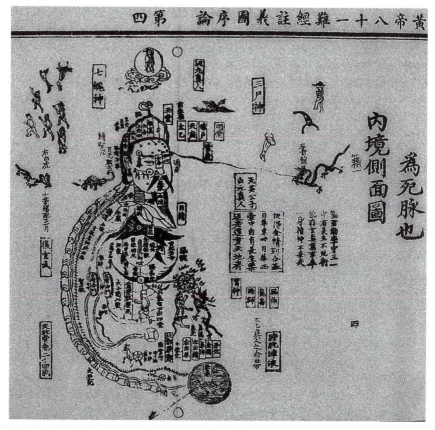

This fifteenth-century Chinese woodblock illustration depicts the internal topography, or landscape (*neijing*), of the human body. The *neijing* illustrations reflect Taoist medico-alchemical concepts of the body, the relationship between the microcosm and the macrocosm, and the quest to prolong life and attain immortality. (Wellcome Library, London)

dynasty (206 B.C.E.–220 C.E.) and was first expressed in the *Huangdi Neijing* (*The Yellow Emperor's Classic of Internal Medicine*). Within this philosophy, the fundamental concept for Chinese medicine is the theory of yin and yang. Yin-yang theory conceives the universe as being composed of a series of paired opposing aspects, such as male and female, light and dark, sun and moon, summer and winter, or heaven and earth. In addition to creating opposition, the aspects of yin and yang are also considered to be united and interdependent, for neither can exist without the other, each contains elements of the other, and they can in fact transform into one another. The body, then, functions in a state of dynamic, ebb-and-flow equilibrium, whereby yin and yang flourish together and vivify each other to maintain health. When this fluctuating state of equilibrium becomes disturbed, depending on whether there is an excess or deficiency in either yin or yang, different illnesses will occur. This concept is expressed in the *Huangdi Neijing* where the physician Ch'i Po explains,

> When Yang is stronger the body is hot, the pores are closed and the people begin to pant; they become boisterous and coarse and whether one looks up or down no perspiration appears. People become feverish (hot), their gums are dry and give trouble, the stomach is affected and people die of constipation. When yang is stronger people can endure winter but they cannot endure summer.
>
> When yin is stronger the body is cold and perspiration appears regularly all over the body. People see their fate clearly; they tremble with fear and get chilled. When they are chilled their spirits become rebellious. Their full stomachs can no longer digest and they die. When yin is stronger people can endure summer but they cannot endure winter.
>
> Thus, yin and yang alternate, their victories vary and so does the character of their diseases. (Veith 1972, 115–121)

The system of correspondences uniting the body with the cosmos is also based on the theory of the *wu xing* (the "five phases" or "five elements"). This theory explains that everything in the universe is composed of the motion and change of the five elements (wood, fire, earth, metal, and water). The motions or phases of the elements allow each to create another in a cycle with water generating wood, wood generating fire, fire generating earth, earth generating metal, and, finally, metal generating water. At the same time, each element is restrained or opposed by another, so that water is contained by earth, while fire is extinguished by water (Figure 1.2).

The elements of the *wu xing* are also understood as existing within a series of systematic correspondences to provide a holistic understanding of the relationship between man and nature. Some of these correspondences are shown in Table 1.1.

According to these correspondences, each of the organs relates to a different element, so that an illness in one organ can be expressed in terms of the five elements. Likewise, the systematic correspondences indicate points for treatment that can restore the harmonious balance of the cycle of relationships in the body that is necessary for the maintenance of health. So, for example, an individual with a flushed face and rapid pulse might be diagnosed as having excess heart fire, so the doctor might seek to nourish the kidneys (water) in order to restrain

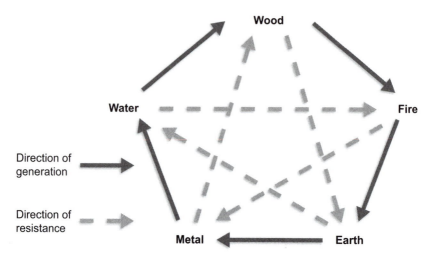

**Figure 1.2** The *wu xing*, or Five Phases.

**Table 1.1** The systematic correspondences of man and nature

| Elements | Seasons | Direction | *Zang* Organs | Six *Fu* Organs | Sense Organs | Emotions |
|---|---|---|---|---|---|---|
| Wood | Spring | East | Liver | Gallbladder | Eyes | Anger |
| Fire | Summer | South | Heart | Small intestine and the "three burning spaces" | Tongue | Joy |
| Earth | Late summer | Middle | Spleen | Stomach | Mouth | Thought |
| Metal | Autumn | West | Lungs | Large intestine | Nose | Sorrow |
| Water | Winter | North | Kidneys | Urinary bladder | Ear | Fear |

the heart and resist the excess fire through the use of medicines or other means. Or, a patient with a deficiency of the kidneys might be treated with medicines to promote the kidneys directly or, better yet, with medicines to strengthen the lungs, which in turn serve to nourish the kidneys according to the cycle of the five elements.

The yin-yang and *wu xing* theories have many similarities, and they are applied together in the process of diagnosing and treating patients. Both rely on an understanding of the need to maintain a balance in the body and explain how a doctor would need to go about either purging or nourishing different aspects of the body in order to restore a healthy equilibrium in sick patients. These theoretical systems also overlay the more anatomical understanding of the body's organs. Traditional Chinese medicine divides the body's internal organs into the five yin organs (*zang*, or viscera) and the six yang organs (*fu*, or bowels) according to their physiological functions. *Zang* organs (liver, heart, spleen, lungs, and kidneys) are responsible for generating and storing, while the *fu* organs (gallbladder, small intestine, stomach, large intestine, urinary bladder, and the "three burning spaces") have the power of eliminating wastes from the body. The *zang* and *fu* organs also fit within the *wu xing* theory, with each organ corresponding to a specific phase or element, thus further tying them into the theoretical model for understanding health and illness (see Table 1.1).

Chinese medical theory also distinguishes certain vital fluids that flow through the body, the most important being *qi* (chee) and blood. The concept of *qi* originated as early as the Spring and Autumn and the Warring States periods (770–221 B.C.E.). Initially, *qi* seems to have had the meaning of a "vapor" or "breath" associated with life but was increasingly recognized as the vital principle (sometimes translated as "energy") that flows through the body. Different types of *qi* (classified according to their composition, the organ in the body with which they are associated, and their physiological function) are responsible for promoting growth; nourishing, warming, and stimulating the organs; and protecting against external influences by regulating the openings of the body through which excretion and secretion of fluids occur. Blood, the other fundamental fluid in the body, serves to nourish and moisten the body. It is primarily composed of nutritional *qi* and it is also regulated by the *qi*. Both *qi* and blood are supposed to flow through meridians or pathways, which connect all of the organs and limbs of the body. The harmonious movement of these fluids, especially *qi*, is deemed necessary for health; obstructions or stagnation leading to accumulation of either fluid in a part of the body leads to disease.

According to this theoretical system, individuals must maintain the harmonious functioning of their bodies by regulating their diet, physical activity, and their emotional state. Extremes in any of these areas would lead to an unhealthy imbalance in the yin-yang, *wu xing*, or the flow of *qi*. In addition to individual behavior, a number of external factors might also cause disease. Traditional Chinese medicine categorizes the environmental or climactic factors that contribute to disease as the "six excesses" (wind, cold, summer heat, dampness, dryness, and fire). In normal conditions the environmental factors (referred to as the "six *qi*") are not harmful and are even important for normal health, but when the climate changes rapidly, or in abnormal or extreme conditions, they are called the "six excesses" that can invade the body to cause illness. Thus, as with the Hippocratic and Ayurvedic traditions, Chinese medical theory recognizes the close interaction between the body (microcosm) and the universe (macrocosm).

## HEALTH AND SOCIAL WELL-BEING

Reflecting on her good fortune in her old age, Adad-guppi, the mother of the Babylonian king Nabonidus (556–539 B.C.E.), thanked the moon-god for her long and comfortable life:

> He [Sin, the moon-god] added (to my life) many days (and) years of happiness and kept me alive . . . one hundred and four happy years (spent) in that piety which Sin, the king of all gods, has planted in my heart. My eyesight was good (to the end of my life), my hearing excellent, my hands and feet were sound, my words well chosen, food and drink agreed with me, my health was fine and my mind happy. I saw my great-great-grandchildren, up to the fourth generation, in good health and (thus) had my fill of old age. (Oppenheim 1969, 561)

Adad-guppi's testimony indicates that she did not see her health as only a biological state, but understood it in the context of her relationship to her god, her family, and her own emotions. This broader concept of health would necessitate the balancing of one's body, as well as one's emotions, and spiritual and social connectedness.

Although the premodern healing traditions we have reviewed developed concepts to identify and classify specific diseases, they mostly viewed health as existing on a continuum, requiring careful efforts to maintain equilibrium in the body. Within these systems, health was not merely the absence of disease, and people did not consider medical advice only when they were sick. Rather, the individual needed continually to be aware of environmental factors as well as the influence of diet and regimen on his current bodily state and take appropriate actions to regulate his activities accordingly in order to safeguard his health. Furthermore, these systems expected that people consider their emotions and their relations to gods, family, and society. Disease processes in the body would certainly play a factor in determining individual well-being, and physicians would have a role in helping to restore health, but the more holistic concepts of health considered here place great emphasis on the part played by individuals in balancing aspects of their physical, mental, and spiritual lives. In later chapters, we will consider these important aspects of health and well-being.

# CHAPTER 2

# Education and Training: Learned and Non-Learned

A wide variety of medical practitioners coexisted in most premodern societies. Anyone could peddle cures or offer treatments part-time, in addition to performing his other occupational duties, but others might seek to make a living solely by offering medical care. In most cases, practitioners were trained through some form of apprenticeship, or acquired their knowledge through practice. Over time, a written medical tradition developed in many premodern societies, suggesting that the body of knowledge associated with the theory and practice of medicine was deemed sufficiently complex and extensive to merit being recorded in texts. Not all healers would necessarily be literate or have access to the written medical tradition, but those whose medical education was complemented by their access to the medical books might distinguish themselves by claiming to have a more sophisticated understanding of health and disease. As a result, a hierarchy of medical practitioners developed in many cultures in which those physicians, whose education included having access to the learned and increasingly theoretical textual medical tradition, were elevated above the majority of other doctors and health care providers, trained solely through apprenticeship or experience in practice. For this reason, it is crucial to examine the rise of written medical traditions in the different cultures we are considering in order to understand the impact learned medicine had on the methods of medical education and the knowledge healers might be expected to possess.

## MEDICAL LEARNING IN THE ANCIENT NEAR EAST

### Mesopotamia

Surviving sources on Mesopotamian medicine (ca. 3000–300 B.C.E.) are mostly written in the cuneiform ("wedge-shaped") writing system, inscribed on clay tablets that were baked for preservation. In total, we have fewer than one thousand tablets or fragments of tablets on medical subjects, and modern scholars must often assemble the fragments as though piecing together a jigsaw puzzle. Because many of the medical texts survive in multiple copies, scholars can see that they underwent constant changes as they were edited, compiled with other texts and copied through the years, suggesting that the Mesopotamian authors continued to modify them based on their own experiences in practice.

The vast majority of surviving tablets come from a single trove, the library of Ashurbanipal (669–629 B.C.E.), the last great king of Assyria, which was destroyed when the invading Medes and Chaldeans invaded the royal city of Nineveh in 612 B.C.E. Ashurbanipal boasted that he had assembled a collection of texts on the three paths to healing: through the use of drugs, operating with the brass knife, and through the prescriptions of the sorcerers. Thus, although they represent sources from a single find, it is clear that Ashurbanipal felt his collection represented a fairly complete coverage of the medical writings of his day and it included copies of much older texts, some perhaps extending back to originals first produced in the third millennium B.C.E.

Most of the surviving medical texts are lists of prescriptions, including both herbal remedies and healing incantations. Others offer collections of case histories arranged under headings that might give some indication of the condition to be treated (e.g., "if the hand of a ghost seizes on a man . . ." or "if a woman gives birth to a child with . . ." or "if a man is affected in the lungs . . ."), which would be followed by suggested remedies. In addition to these shorter texts one finds a few longer, more sophisticated medical works, such as the *Treatise of Medical Diagnoses and Prognoses*, which consists of forty tablets organized around the recognition of certain signs that should be observed when determining the cause of the illness and foretelling its future course in the patient. This text opens with a discussion of the omens that might be observed on the way to the sick person's home, followed by a list of the signs (from head to foot) the doctor should watch for in the patient's body. Later sections cover the daily progress of several conditions with the intent of providing a prognosis, and the methods of treating specific conditions (whether by incantations or herbal remedies), with a final section specifically devoted to the diseases of women and pregnancy.

The sources reveal that there were three main kinds of healers in Mesopotamian societies: the *baru* (seer), trained in the art of divination; the *ashipu* (exorcist), a priest who treated sick people as one of his many religious duties; and the *asu* (physician), a priest devoted to treating the sick with charms, drugs, and surgical cures. Rather than competing with each other for patients, it seems that each of these healers served a particular function in the healing process and that they would work together to bring about the cure of the patient. This point is clearly made in one letter written to the king in which a sick official requests that the king, "appoint at my side an *ashipu* [exorcist] and an *asu* [physician] . . . may they perform the ceremonies on my behalf" (Sigerist 1951, 431). The *asu*, however, was most specifically dedicated to the treatment of the sick. In a hymn praising Gula, one of the primary healing deities, the goddess describes herself as an *asu*, providing some sense of the range of activities with which the *asu* might be associated:

> I am a physician, I can heal,
> I carry around all [healing] herbs, I drive away disease,
> I gird myself with the leather bag containing health-giving incantations.
> I carry around texts which bring recovery,
> I give cures to mankind.
> My pure dressing alleviates the wound,
> My soft bandage relieves the sick. (Lambert 1967, 121)

We should first note that the *asu* was known for his textual learning. Beyond that, the *asu* was also associated with a variety of therapeutic devices including herbal cures, incantations, and wound dressings. From other sources, such as the Code of Hammurabi, a listing of 282 laws engraved on a stone block in the first half of the eighteenth century B.C.E., we know that the *asu* was also the healer responsible for providing a variety of surgical operations. Thus, textual learning and practical experience together define the *asu*'s education.

As members of the priestly classes, the *ashipu* and the *asu* would have been among the most well-educated people in Mesopotamian society and would have trained within the major temples, where they would have learned the skills necessary for reading and writing the cuneiform script. In this context, their medical training probably required the study of the written sources of learned medicine, and having access to that written tradition no doubt served as a significant distinguishing feature of these health care providers, establishing their credentials as learned men. Some evidence suggests that medical learning was protected as a form of secret knowledge that was not to be spread widely outside this community of medical scholars. For example, several texts end with instructions such as, "May he who knows instruct him who knows. And may he who knows not, not read this" and "He who does not keep the secret will not remain in health." Such efforts to control access to medical learning reinforce the idea that the written learned tradition of medicine was a central component of the identity of these healing classes. Although there is no evidence of formal apprenticeship programs for the *baru, ashipu,* or *asu,* it is possible that part of their training would involve developing their skills through practice under the guidance of an experienced teacher. The efforts to control access to written medical learning and the fact that practical medical training through apprenticeship receives little attention in the texts suggest that access to the written medical sources was considered the central component of the identity of these health care professionals.

## Egypt

Our knowledge of ancient Egyptian medicine (covering the period from ca. 3150–332 B.C.E.) is based largely on roughly a dozen important medical papyri produced between 1900 B.C.E. and 300 B.C.E. These papyri, usually written in the hieratic script (similar to the hieroglyphic writing system), if translated and printed, would comprise just over two hundred pages of text today and likely represent only a small fraction of the medical works produced in ancient Egypt, which have otherwise been lost through the ravages of time. The earliest of these papyri, the Kahun papyrus, produced around 1825 B.C.E., is a fragmented and relatively short document that focuses exclusively on diseases of women. The Ebers papyrus (ca. 1500 B.C.E.), a compendium of several shorter medical treatises, seemingly arranged at random, is by far the longest medical papyrus. It includes several remedies for specific medical conditions, including eye diseases, urinary difficulties, dental concerns, crocodile bites, and other conditions that are more difficult to define such as *wekhedu* (which could either mean "pain" or refer to a substance thought to cause putrefaction and decomposition within the body).

The written sources indicate at least three categories of people were involved in healing in ancient Egypt: priests, magicians, and *swnw* (typically pronounced "sewnew" and translated as either "physician" or "doctor"). Although it is now clear that priests did not restrict their healing to merely saying prayers and *swnw* were equally likely to prescribe magical cures, it does appear that the *swnw* were known mostly for their naturalistic medical theories concerning the body and disease, the application of physical treatments, and the preparation of pharmaceutical remedies. The phrase, "placing of the hands," is commonly associated with *swnw* in the medical papyri, perhaps indicating that they were specifically known for hands-on diagnosis and treatment. Many *swnw* were identified as focusing on particular areas of practice, (e.g., doctors of the abdomen or doctors of the eyes), suggesting a high degree of medical specialization.

The Edwin Smith surgical papyrus (ca. 1550 B.C.E.), the oldest surviving surgical text in the world and second longest of the Egyptian medical papyri, provides perhaps the best sense of the practice of a *swnw*. Unlike most other medical papyri that simply present a compilation of remedies, it is organized as an instruction book listing a number of different medical cases with helpful advice on how the *swnw* would arrive at a diagnosis and determine treatment. It presents each case in four parts: the title or concise description of the condition, the examination of the patient and the symptoms, the diagnosis and prognosis, and the treatment. The diagnosis is typically followed by one of three prognoses, indicating the *swnw*'s opinion as to the outcome: "An ailment which I will treat," "An ailment with which I will contend," or "An ailment not to be treated." One entry (likely describing a case of tetanus) reads as follows:

> *Title*: Instructions for a gaping wound in his head, extending to the bone, penetrating the *tepau* of his skull.
>
> *First Examination*: . . . You should then probe his wound though he shudders greatly. You should then cause him to lift his face. It is painful for him to open his mouth. His heart beats too slowly (or weakly) for speech. You observe his saliva falling from his lips but not falling completely. He discharges blood from his two nostrils and from his two ears. He suffers stiffness in his neck. He does not find he can look at his two shoulders and his breast.
>
> *First diagnosis and prognosis*: You shall say concerning him . . . the cord of his mandible is contracted; he discharges blood from his two nostrils and from his two ears; and he suffers stiffness in his neck—an ailment with which I will contend.

*First treatment*: As soon as you find that man, the cord of his mandibles and his jaws are contracted, you should cause one to make for him something hot until he is comfortable and his mouth opens. You should then bind it with oil and honey until you know he has reached a decisive point.

*Second examination*: If you find in that man that his flesh has developed heat under the wound, which is in the *tepau* of his skull. That man, he has developed toothache under that wound. You put your hand on him and you find his brow is wet with sweat. The muscles of his neck are taut, his face is flushed. . . . The odor of . . . his head is like the excrement of small cattle. His mouth is bound, his two eyebrows drawn, his face is as if he was weeping.

*Second diagnosis and prognosis*: You shall then say concerning him . . . he has developed toothache; his mouth is bound; he suffers stiffness of his neck—an ailment not to be treated. (Nunn 1996, 181–182)

The medical papyri were undoubtedly used for teaching purposes, but this would require that the *swnw* be literate. Those young and literate *swnw*, who possessed a copy of a medical papyrus, would have been able to use them in their studies, while the less fortunate might have had access to written medical knowledge through the *per ankh* (House of Life), a scriptorium where books were compiled. Otherwise, medical practice appears to have been taught from father to son through a system of apprenticeship. Numerous funeral stela, gravestones, indicate that sons followed the professions of their fathers in ancient Egypt, and one Greek historian considering Egyptian healers suggested that medicine was the one profession where children were required to follow in their parents' footsteps. Therefore, though it is likely that the *swnw* was often a member of the learned, literate class who would have access to the written medical texts, some *swnw* may have only been trained through apprenticeship, learning the craft of medicine by practicing with their fathers.

## MEDICAL LEARNING IN THE ANCIENT GREEK AND ROMAN WORLD

### Hippocratic Medicine

The Hippocratic Corpus, which is a collection of about sixty medical texts written between 420 and 350 B.C.E. and attributed to Hippocrates of Cos, represent the earliest Greek writings on medical subjects. Although it is likely that some of these texts were written by the historical Hippocrates, scholars continue to debate which ones might have genuinely been written by him. It is clear that the texts of the Hippocratic Corpus were written in different Greek dialects and often present contradictory theoretical opinions and cures and thus the same individual could not have written them all. They are united, however, by a shared interest in establishing a naturalistic, rational system for explaining disease and cures, without reference to divine or magical interventions. Furthermore, they identify those healers who followed this more naturalistic approach to medicine as *iatroi* (sing. *iatros*), or doctors.

The books of the Hippocratic Corpus attempt to do many different things. Some seek to justify a particular theoretical viewpoint regarding the practice of medicine (e.g., *On Ancient Medicine* and *The Art of Medicine*) or offer a theoretical explanation for the humoral causes of disease in the body (e.g., *On the Nature of Man*). By contrast, other texts focus more on providing detailed observations of the symptoms and course of diseases in patients (e.g., *Epidemics*), explain the practice of diagnosis and prognosis (e.g., *On Prognosis*), offer advice for how to regulate diet and regimen to maintain health (e.g., *A Regimen for Health*), or discuss certain kinds of surgical operations (e.g., *On Head Wounds* and *On Joints*). Still other texts offer opinions on how an *iatros* should behave or appear to have been aimed at teaching (e.g., the *Oath* and the *Aphorisms*). Therefore, although the Hippocratic Corpus shares a naturalistic approach to disease and healing, the works offer a diverse array of opinions on the kinds of knowledge necessary for practice.

The *iatroi*, who followed the doctrines in the newly forming written medical tradition, would practice alongside an array of religious healers, midwives, bonesetters, and folk practitioners. But the *iatroi* were a diverse group themselves, whose writings suggest some significant theoretical and practical differences, making it impossible to generalize about the expected requirements for training and practice. Indeed, there were no medical regulations, and those who sought to practice medicine were not required to undergo any examinations or to adhere to a specific set of expectations. Even the *Oath*, perhaps the most famous Hippocratic text, represents only one opinion as to the minimum expectations for the behavior of medical practitioners, and it is not reflected in other books from the Corpus. In general, a Hippocratic *iatros* likely practiced as an itinerant healer, traveling from town to town, offering his services for a fee, in competition with a diverse range of other healers. In this context, it appears that perhaps the main skill the *iatros* could offer to distinguish himself from others was his claim to a theoretical understanding of the disease process combined with an ability to diagnose a particular illness and offer an accurate prognosis for its course (abilities emphasized in several texts from the Corpus) that would convince a potential client of his abilities.

Most *iatroi* were probably trained through a system of apprentice-ship, where fathers would teach their craft to their sons or train those from outside the family for a fee. The *Oath* gives some indication of the expectations of an apprentice, who was expected to swear to follow his teacher as he would his father and "to give a share of precepts and oral instruction and all the other learning to my sons and to the sons of him who has instructed me and to pupils who have signed the covenant and have taken an oath according to the medical law, but to no one else" (Edelstein 1967, 6). No reference is made to the necessity of having access to a written tradition, but students would be expected to learn certain precepts through oral instruction. In some cases, the precepts were likely presented as we find them in the *Aphorisms*, as a series of brief, memorable statements that offered guidance for diagnosis, prog-nosis, and treatment. For example, the first aphorism emphasizes the many things the *iatros* should take into consideration when practicing his craft: "Life is short, the art long; opportunity is elusive, experiment is dangerous and judgment is difficult. It is not enough for the physi-cian to do what is necessary, but the patient and the attendants must do their part as well, and circumstances must be favorable" (Chadwick and Mann 1950, 206). Later aphorisms offer more direct advice, relat-ing that the elderly can handle fasting better than the young; that fluid diets are especially beneficial in cases of fever; or that pregnant women should not be given drugs after the seventh month of gestation.

### Galen and the Hippocratic Tradition

As the body of written medical knowledge grew, many came to believe that a physician should be well versed in the theoretical principles it conveyed. One of those who held that physicians should be trained through reading texts was Galen of Pergamum (129–ca. 216 c.e.). He was born to a wealthy family in the Greek-speaking part of the Roman Empire and received a typical upper-class education, which emphasized the importance of philosophical learning. Fairly early in his life, he decided to pursue a career in medicine and went to study in Alexandria, Egypt, the most famous center of medical learning in his day, where he studied the texts of learned Greek medicine. He returned to Pergamum, where he served as doctor to gladiators for several years before heading to Rome to further his career and enhance his reputation. Galen regularly engaged in public (often heated) dis-putations with rival doctors in Rome, earning their animosity, but he also achieved several successful cures and soon could claim a clientele drawn from the highest levels of Roman society. By 168, he became doctor to the emperor and held this position with successive emperors until his death. Galen's meteoric rise is testimony to his skills as a healer, but also to the growing success of the learned Greek tradition within the Roman world.

In addition to his successful medical practice, Galen also wrote extensively on medicine and over 350 works confirmed as written by him survive today, more than from any other writer on medicine from antiquity. He wrote extensively on the theories and methods of diagnosis through the pulse and other signs and on how to link these observations to knowledge about the underlying physiological and pathological processes of the body. In order to make these connections, he emphasized the need for physicians to understand human anatomy and the functioning of the different structures in the body. He wrote extensive commentaries on the books of the Hippocratic Corpus, smoothing over their contradictions, emphasizing certain points and de-emphasizing others. In the process, Galen explained the Hippocratic Corpus so as to make it appear as a unified whole, and it was his interpretation that would guide later people's understanding of those texts into the twentieth century. Together, Galen's medical writings drew upon the texts of the learned Greek tradition and reformed them into a cohesive, systematic, philosophical tradition that would shape medical learning in the West for several centuries. Furthermore, Galen wrote about the various therapeutic methods (including diet, drug lore, bloodletting, and other forms of surgery) and the theories that would govern their application in practice. Taken together, Galen's medical writings explored the entire range of learned medicine available in his day and impressed his stamp upon it.

In his works, Galen also established very high expectations for the range of knowledge a doctor should command, declaring that both textual learning and experience in practice were essential for the ideal physician. He argued that the ideal physician should be highly educated and learned in Greek philosophy (including the works of Aristotle, Plato, and the Stoic philosophers) as well as the written medical tradition, since he maintained that philosophic reasoning should guide the practice of the healer at the bedside. At the same time, Galen believed the physician needed to be an attentive observer who could learn through experience how to diagnose a patient's illness based on a wide variety of symptoms and know which remedies were especially appropriate in different cases. Although many Romans were doubtful of the value of text-based medical knowledge (favoring traditional, empirical remedies), Galen helped to shape the written medical tradition that would define learned medical practice in the later Islamic and European worlds.

## MEDICAL LEARNING IN INDIA: THE WRITTEN TRADITION OF AYURVEDA

### The Origin of the Ayurvedic Medical Texts

Ayurveda (literally "knowledge for longevity") has its roots in the oral traditions passed on by practicing healers from the Vedic period (ca. 1500–500 B.C.E.), including the rational or naturalistic medical knowledge of the *sramanas*, wandering ascetics who pursued knowledge of the natural world for its own sake, and the magical healing of the *bhishaj*, healers known for their incantations and spells aimed at curing specific ailments and also for making amulets and talismans from plants and other substances that could ward off demons and malign spells in order to bring about a cure. The transition of these oral traditions into written form came about mostly as a result of the work of Buddhist monks. Shortly after the rise of Buddhism in the sixth century B.C.E., Buddhist ascetics (monks and nuns) began to organize into monastic communities called *sanghas*. These communities encouraged wanderers to visit and engage in debates over a variety

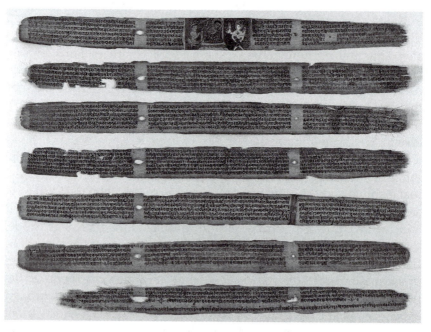

These passages from a copy of the *Susruta Samhita*, one of the foundational texts of Ayurvedic medicine, are written on palm leaves. This version was produced in the eighteenth or nineteenth century, reflecting the longstanding value of this medical book. (Digital Image © 2012 Museum Associates/LACMA. Licensed by Art Resource, NY)

of subjects, including medicine. The *sanghas* quickly became centers for medical learning, where Buddhist monks, starting in the mid-fifth century B.C.E., began to collect, organize, and write down the content of the oral tradition, creating the central texts of Ayurvedic medicine. As a result, it is difficult to know exactly when the earliest texts of the Ayurveda were first composed in written form, although estimates for the different texts suggest dates between 1000 and 500 B.C.E., and even then, the texts continued to be revised and added to until the fourth or fifth century C.E., making it difficult to speak of dates of composition with much certainty.

The earliest of the Ayurvedic texts, the *Caraka Samhita*, appears to have been written down around the second century C.E., although it compiles a number of seemingly disparate materials that were much older. It consists of 120 chapters divided into eight parts including sections on the theoretical classification of diseases, pharmacology, anatomy, and embryology. It also includes more practically oriented sections on diagnosis, prognosis, and therapy for specific diseases. In general, it reflects the more naturalistic medical tradition of the *sramanas*, but it also contains some magical and religious therapies, indicating that it draws upon multiple sources of Vedic medicine. The other early Ayurvedic text, the *Susruta Samhita*, like the *Caraka*, includes passages that reflect a much earlier origin, but it appears to have been written down in its current form around the fourth century C.E. The *Susruta* is divided into six large sections and covers similar material to the *Caraka* (theories of pathology, embryology, and pharmacy, as well as discussions of various methods of diagnosis, prognosis, and treatment, and some explanations for managing diseases ascribed to demonic attacks). Unlike the *Caraka*, however, the *Susruta* also provides extensive coverage of the theory and practice of surgery and discusses methods of surgical training.

Since the *Caraka* and *Susruta* draw upon a number of earlier sources they are not clearly organized and sometimes include conflicting material. Later, in the fifth century C.E., the *Astangahrdaya* (*The Heart of Medicine*), ascribed to Vagbhata, was composed with the intention of synthesizing the disordered and conflicting material found in the previous texts to create a systematic presentation of the principles of Ayurvedic medicine. Indeed, it would eclipse the *Caraka* and *Susruta* to become the most widely translated and circulated Ayurvedic text and the core text for Ayurvedic medical education into the nineteenth century. Together, the *Caraka*, the *Susruta*, and *The Heart of Medicine* are known as the *Brihat Trayi* ("the greater triad") to distinguish them from the later three medical texts known together as the *Laghu Trayi* ("lesser triad"): the *Madhava Nidana* (composed between 700 and 1100 c.e.), the *Sarangadhara Samhita* (fourteenth century c.e.), and the *Bhavaprakasha* (sixteenth century c.e.). The *Laghu Trayi* and other medical works from the eighth through sixteenth centuries reveal the growing consolidation of Ayurvedic medicine and devote increasing attention to the classification of diseases, to new methods of diagnosis (including pulse lore), to descriptions of newly discovered sexually transmitted diseases (including syphilis), and to the growing use of metal and mineral substances in pharmacy.

## Medical Education

Medical education in the Vedic period was based in an oral tradition; teachers would sing the hymns or recite the verses from the Vedas or medical collections and the student would be expected to learn them by heart. This explains why written versions of these works were sometimes not produced until centuries after the oral "text" had been in circulation and also why they existed in mostly verse form. The *Caraka* and *Susruta* both reflect this method of teaching, being framed explicitly as accounts of a teacher passing along his knowledge to a single student. To this end, they offer advice for teachers on elocution, how to recite the words of the verses, and traditional lore clearly and properly, and also admonish the teacher to provide useful commentary upon the materials to help the student's comprehension and memorization. Students were expected to hone their theoretical knowledge by regularly engaging in discussions by means of which they could clarify their understanding of the materials and develop their eloquence. The true doctor, by these accounts, would be a man of learning eager to seek out new knowledge for its own sake.

Medical students did not only learn theoretical precepts. The author of the *Susruta* declared that "he who is only trained in theory, but is not experienced in practice knows not what he should do when he has a patient and behaves as foolishly as a youth upon a battlefield. On the other hand, a physician who is educated practically, but not in theory, will not earn the respect of better men" (Kutumbiah 1962, xlix). Therefore, students were also expected to assist their teacher in the treatment of patients, to help in the preparation of medicaments, and to practice their skills with the tools of the trade. Indeed, the Susruta suggests that students practice their surgical skills by working on pieces of wood, dried gourds, fruit, and dead animals.

From the fifth century b.c.e. onward, the Buddhist *sanghas* began to play an increasingly important role in medical education serving as centers where wandering ascetics interested in pursuing an education in the arts, sciences, traditional Brahmanism, and also medicine might gather to engage in intellectual debate. The role of Buddhist monasteries as centers for education was expanded toward the end of the Gupta dynasty (mid-sixth century C.E.) when the "greater monasteries" (*mahavihara*) started to develop a core curriculum. A Chinese Buddhist pilgrim visiting the *mahavihara* at Nalanda in the early seventh century C.E. noted that it drew students from all over and that they would study core subjects including the five sciences (*vidya*) and the major works of Buddhist philosophy. Medicine was one of the five sciences and therefore all students would study the texts of the classical Ayurvedic tradition alongside the other important Vedic texts. As a result, by the end of the seventh century C.E., Ayurvedic medicine was established as a central component of the curriculum as one of the five sciences taught in Buddhist monasteries and as Buddhism spread to other parts of Asia, the Ayurvedic medical system spread with it.

## MEDICAL LEARNING IN CHINA

### Foundations of Traditional Chinese Medicine

The most renowned early text of the Chinese medical tradition, the *Huangdi Neijing* (*The Yellow Emperor's Classic of Internal Medicine*), was likely written by several authors, bringing together earlier medical materials, including writings on demonic and magical medicine, and coalesced into its final form during the Han dynasty (206 B.C.E.–220 C.E.), probably just prior to the first century C.E. The *Huangdi Neijing* consists of two parts, the *Suwen* (*The Basic Questions*) and the *Lingshu* (*The Divine Pivot*). The *Suwen* is presented as a dialogue between the Yellow Emperor, Huangdi, and his ministers and provides the fundamental theories concerning anatomy, physiology, and methods of diagnosis and treatment. It includes discussions of medical concepts of *yin* and *yang*, the circulation of *qi* in the body, the theory of the correspondence of the "five phases" (*wu xing*), and theories about the organs and their functions. The *Lingshu*, by contrast, is more narrowly focused on acupuncture and moxibustion therapy as a means of regulating the flow of *qi* through the body's twelve meridians. The *Huangdi Neijing*, therefore, represents a move toward providing a naturalistic theoretical system for understanding health and disease (in contrast to the belief in magical, demonic medicine prevalent in earlier periods) and it would quickly become the foundational text for traditional Chinese medicine.

Numerous texts from this early period, including the *Huangdi Neijing* and the *Nanjing* (*Classic on Difficult Medical Problems*), reveal the development of the theory and practice of acupuncture as a form of treatment. Other texts, like those by Zhang Zhongjing (150–219 C.E.), one of the most famous physicians from the later Han dynasty, were especially concerned with the methods of diagnosis and how to match treatment to the theoretical explanations for disease. In his two texts, the *Shang-hanlun* (*On Cold-induced Diseases*) and *Jingui Yaolue* (*Synopsis of the Golden Bookcase*) Zhang focused his attention on the classification of diseases according to which of the meridians or viscera they affected and placed heavy emphasis on linking the observed symptoms to the underlying part of the body being affected. In this way, he sought to unite clinical observation with the theoretical understanding and the theory of systematic correspondence of anatomy and physiology. Zhang's text and others also reveal the development of a detailed theory of drug therapy, explaining how medicines should be prescribed according to the theory of systematic correspondence to treat the specific causes of the disease in the body. Thus, the foundation for the theoretical precepts of traditional Chinese medicine was largely laid by the end of the third century C.E.

### The Rise of Formal Medical Education

The *Huangdi Neijing* offers insight into the methods of medical education up through the Han dynasty. In this work, the medical master, Huang Di, the legendary Yellow Emperor, is depicted teaching the theory and practice of medicine to a small group of students. The Yellow Emperor emphasizes the importance of referring to the classical medical texts as a basis for instruction, but also expects students to acquire empirical knowledge by assisting their masters in the treatment of patients. Following this model, individual physicians would take on apprentices and train them in the art of medicine through a discussion of key texts and practice at the bedside. Although education was done on an individual basis, records from the Zhou dynasty (1045–256 B.C.E.) reveal the early existence of state-administered medical examinations for physicians, although it is not clear how effectively they were enforced. However, there is no indication that they were tied to state-administered medical education.

The move toward governmental supervision over medical education was most pronounced in the Tang dynasty (618–907 C.E.). Medicine had previously become one of the subjects taught at the Imperial Academy, which oversaw the education of civil servants, but under the Tang the Imperial Bureau of Medicine was established and divided the teaching of medicine into four sections: internal medicine, acupuncture, massage (which included the treatment of wounds), and incantations. Furthermore, a separate department within the Bureau was made responsible for maintaining botanical gardens and teaching the subject of pharmacology. From the beginning, students studied the classical medical texts and more organized recent summaries, including the *Huangdi Neijing*, the works of Zhang Zhongjing, and the *Zhenjiu Jiayijing* (*The ABC of Acupuncture and Moxibustion*), the central text on the practice of acupuncture.

Chinese medical education underwent further profound changes starting in the eleventh century C.E. with the rise of technologies for woodblock printing, which allowed for the wider diffusion of medical learning. Under the Song dynasty (960–1279 C.E. ), the Bureau for the Re-editing of Medical Books was created in 1057 for the purpose of collecting, editing, and printing the important medical texts from the preceding 1,000 years. The first books printed by this bureau (in order) were the *Suwen* from the *Huangdi Neijing*, the *Shang-hanlun* and the *Jingui Yaolue* by Zhang Zhongjing, and the *Zhenjiu Jiayijing*. At the same time that medical texts were being brought to a wider audience through printing, the Imperial Bureau of Medicine supervised the establishment of medical schools in each of the prefectures in China and reformed the medical curriculum and examination system. Medical education revolved around the study of the previously named texts, alongside the *Nanjing*, the *Zhubing Yuanhoulun* (*Treatise on the Causes and Symptoms of Maladies*) by Chao Yuanfang (fl. sixth–seventh century C.E.), and the pharmacology text by Sun Simiao (581–682), the *Qianjin Yaofang* (*Prescriptions of the Thousand Ounces of Gold*).

Students in the medical schools during the Song dynasty and later would be tested both orally and clinically, and in both cases they were expected to be able to display their knowledge of the theoretical medical system and use it to justify their treatments. Exam scores were ranked, and those who scored in the highest rank would be given official appointments as teachers and asked to write medical books; those in the second rank would be given licenses to practice, while students with lower scores were told to study further and take the exam again, or to pursue careers in a different profession. Teachers were also examined each year based upon the success rate of their students, and in the Yuan dynasty (1271–1368 C.E.) two decrees were passed for punishing incompetent or lazy teachers who failed to ensure that their students attend lectures regularly and study the prescribed texts.

In many ways the greater consolidation of medical education also encouraged the development of medical specialization. Increasingly, from the Tang dynasty forward, a number of more narrowly focused medical treatises were produced indicating the increased interest in medical specialties such as pediatrics, gynecology, and obstetrics. The move toward medical specialization in turn led to a fragmentation of Chinese medicine into four main schools of thought during the Yuan dynasty, each of which emphasized different factors in the cause of disease and advocated different methods of treatment. For example, the Hejian school, inaugurated by Liu Wan-su (1110–1200) maintained that disease was largely caused by the elements of fire and heat in the body and therefore founded the "school of cooling" which employed "cold" and bitter medicines to counteract unhealthy heat in the body according to the theoretical framework of systemic correspondences. By contrast, Chang Ts'ung-cheng (1156–1228), founder of a competing school of thought, focused his attention on harmful influences from outside the body as the cause of disease; therefore, Chang aimed at expelling the harmful agents from the body by using a variety of emetics and purgatives to induce sweating, sneezing, salivation, vomiting, and other forms of purgation. Despite their differing opinions on disease causation and treatment, the leaders of each of these schools turned to the same range of ancient medical texts to support their positions. In this way, they testify to the fact that the major elements of traditional Chinese medicine had been established by the classical texts from the previous periods, but they also reveal that Chinese medicine was an extremely dynamic system that continued to evolve and develop in response to new theories and observations in practice.

Those physicians trained in the schools supervised by the Imperial Bureau of Medicine represented a minority of all health care providers in Chinese society, however. They were the elite among medical practitioners and were mostly involved only in treating wealthy patients at court, although some may also have provided charitable medical assistance to the general public at times as well. The majority of people would still seek medical assistance from wise women, itinerant drug sellers, magical or religious healers, or other forms of healers who continued to learn their craft through apprenticeship or in practice, with little or no exposure to the texts of learned medicine.

## MEDICAL LEARNING IN THE ISLAMIC WORLD

### Translation and the Written Tradition of Islamic Medicine

The rise of Islam in the seventh century and its rapid spread from Arabia and the Near East across North Africa and into Spain brought the

Arabic-speaking world into increased contact with outside cultures and new ideas. Cultural exchange as a result of trade with the Byzantine Empire, the Persian Empire, and indirectly with places as far-flung as India and China allowed for rapid influx of new learning back to the Islamic world. Under the patronage of the caliphs in Baghdad, scholars in the late eighth and increasingly in the ninth centuries translated texts from a variety of languages (Syriac, Pahlavi, Sanskrit, and especially Greek) into Arabic. Although the translation effort made available works from many medical traditions, including texts of Ayurvedic medicine, translations of Greek texts were by far the most numerous. Hunayn ibn Ishaq (d. ca. 873 or 877), a Nestorian Christian in southern Iraq known later in the Latin West as Johannitius, was one of the leading figures in this translation movement; he and his circle of colleagues were responsible for translating 129 Galenic medical works into Arabic. As a result, the ninth century stands as a formative period for Islamic medicine that was largely shaped by Greek medical philosophy, and most especially Galen's approach to medicine. The Greek system provided a rationalist foundation to Islamic medicine that would transform the Arab medical beliefs and come to characterize the Islamic physician.

By the tenth century, Islamic scholars shifted their attention from translation efforts to producing new medical scholarship of their own. Some of these early works provided detailed observations on specific diseases and their cures, including Hunayn's *Ten Treatises on the Eye* and *On Smallpox and Measles* by Abu Bakr Muhammad ibn Zakariya al-Razi (d. ca. 925, known as Rhazes in the Latin West). Islamic scholars also wrote more far-reaching, comprehensive medical compendia that covered a wide array of theoretical and practical issues in medicine and attempted to organize the vast materials found in their Greek sources. The *Book for Al-Mansur* (later translated into Latin as the *Liber medicinalis ad almansorem*), written by al-Razi and dedicated to a local Iranian prince, is one example of these compendia. In this text, he divided medicine into "theory" and "practice" and drew upon the Greek tradition to discuss the wide range of knowledge deemed valuable for a learned physician. The *Book for Al-Mansur* was divided into ten books: the first six books covered theoretical subjects including anatomy, physiology, general pathology, and pharmacy, while the last four books covered the practical subjects of diagnosis and therapy (including surgery), with book 9 devoted to discussions of specific diseases arranged from head to foot. Similarly, Abu al-Qasim al-Zahrawi (fl. ca. 1000, known as Albucasis in the Latin West), who worked in Cordoba, Spain, wrote another compendium, *The Arrangement of Medical Knowledge for One Who Is Not Able to Compile a Book for Himself*, drawing upon the Greek authorities. Although he relied heavily on the Greek texts, al-Zahrawi often added to it with testimony from his own personal experience, especially in sections where he covers subjects that received little attention in other sources, such as midwifery. The surgical chapters also reflect his personal innovation and they included numerous illustrations of surgical instruments, in themselves a new addition to the surgical literature. Perhaps the most widely influential of these Islamic medical compendia was the *Canon of Medicine* by Ibn Sina (d. 1037, known as Avicenna in the Latin West). Ibn-Sina's *Canon* attempted to situate medicine within the system of Aristotelian natural philosophy. Unlike the previous compendia by al-Razi, al-Zahrawi, and others, Ibn Sina organized his massive text into five books covering the major tenets of theoretical medicine and emphasizing the distinction between diseases specific to one part of the body and more generalized conditions. He also explained specific forms of treatment for different diseases (including bloodletting, cautery, and surgery) and provided a theoretical discussion of medicinal substance and how to mix compound medicines. The careful and logical arrangement of these materials provided a systematic organization and elaboration to the Greek medical theories, and the *Canon* quickly became one of the preeminent texts of Islamic medicine. Based on this text, Ibn Sina would be recognized in the Latin West as one of the three foremost medical authorities, alongside Galen and Hippocrates.

### Practitioners and Their Training

The rapid expansion of Arabic medical literature in the Islamic world led to the development of a new kind of medical practitioner, the physician, who would be knowledgeable in the theories presented in the learned written tradition. By the tenth century, many scholars wrote about the need to examine and license physicians before they would be allowed to practice. Although these regulations were mainly applied in the large urban centers, and were likely to have been largely unsuccessful at excluding those who did not meet minimum standards from practice, they do indicate a growing belief that a physician should be familiar with the learned written sources and able to discuss the theories presented in them when considering problems of diagnosis and treatment. Although physicians were also expected to have experience with bonesetting, reducing dislocations, cautery, cutting with the knife, and other manual procedures, the emphasis placed on their theoretical knowledge shows that their identity was largely founded on their familiarity with the written medical tradition.

Physicians might come by their knowledge of the written medical tradition in a variety of ways. Some, like Ibn Sina, claimed to have been self-taught by studying the authoritative medical texts for themselves. More often, physicians likely learned their trade through apprenticeship, either with a family member, or another practicing physician. By far the most important space for acquiring a medical education, however, was the hospital. According to Ali ibn al-Abbas al-Majusi (fl. ca. 983, known as Haly Abbas in the Latin West), in his medical compendium, the *Complete Book of the Medical Arts*:

> One of the requirements for the student of this art is that he should be in attendance at the hospitals and the places of the sick; that he consult extensively with the most skilled teachers among the physicians about the patients' situations and circumstances; and that he examine frequently the conditions of the patients and the symptoms apparent in them, calling to mind what he has read about these conditions and what they indicate of good and ill. If he does this, he will reach a high degree of perfection in this art. (Pormann and Savage-Smith 2007, 81)

Based on al-Majusi's description, we see that physicians were expected to be able to readily incorporate their theoretical, textual training into practice at the patient's bedside. Islamic hospitals thus offered an ideal setting in which to study medicine because they brought together learned physicians able to teach the textual tradition and the opportunity to observe a variety of diseases and gain experience with the various means of therapeutics when interacting with the patients.

Although the learned physicians were well regarded for their medical expertise, they represented a small minority of all medical practitioners in the Islamic world. Physicians were more likely to practice in the aristocratic courts, in the hospitals, and in the homes of wealthy patients. However, a wide range of less respectable healers offered their medical services in the marketplace. These lower-status healers were often itinerant, offering a range of specialized services as bonesetters, oculists, or sellers of various remedies, and likely had little, if any, training in the theoretical medical tradition. Judging from the large number of vitriolic attacks against women healers found in the texts of Islamic physicians, it appears that women were especially active as healers in the marketplace, treating not only women and children but also men. One physician even speaks with amazement about the patient who "acquiesces to whatever extravagant measure [the woman healer] might order, consumes whatever she prepares for him, and listens to what she says and obeys her commands more than he obeys the physician. He believes that this woman, despite her lack of intelligence, is more knowledgeable and of sounder opinion than the physician" (Pormann and Savage-Smith 2007, 103). Clearly, this physician believed that his textual training should convey a greater respect and distinguish him from the women healers. This example makes clear, however, that patients would seek out a wide variety of learned and non-learned healers and the limited numbers of learned physicians meant that most people, especially in rural settings, would only be able to turn to the self-taught empiric healers for medical treatment.

## MEDICAL LEARNING IN MEDIEVAL EUROPE

### Translation and the Rise of Universities

As with the Islamic tradition, learned medicine in medieval Europe was built upon the written texts from the Greek medical tradition. For much of the early Middle Ages the majority of those texts were not available in Latin, the language of learning in the West, and few knew how to read Greek. However, the eleventh and twelfth centuries witnessed a dramatic increase in trade and cultural exchange between Western Europe, the Greek East, and the Arab world so that from about 1080 onward, scholars were able to translate both Greek and Arabic medical texts into Latin. The rapid influx of previously unavailable medical scholarship containing a more theoretically sophisticated medical system greatly expanded the amount of learned medical literature available and strengthened the philosophical component of medical knowledge.

The sudden profusion of new medical learning in Latin sparked profound changes in the study and practice of medicine in the West. Since the late tenth century, Salerno, in southern Italy, had been recognized as a center of medical practice, not book learning. Over the course of the twelfth century, however, the Salernitan practitioners were ideally located to take advantage of the newly translated medical literature and they began to incorporate it into their teaching to provide a more theoretical, academic medical education. By the mid-twelfth century, the Salernitan masters had identified a collection of texts, referred to as the *Articella*, which would form the core of the medical curriculum. The *Articella* consisted of five main texts (Johannitius's *Isagoge*, Hippocrates's *Aphorisms* and *Prognosis*, and two short Byzantine treatises on the methods of diagnosis, Theophilus's *On Urines* and Philaretus's *On Pulses*), which were soon supplemented in the curriculum by Galen's *Art of Healing* (known as the *Tegni* or *Microtegni* in the Middle Ages in order to distinguish it from Galen's *Therapeutic Method*, known as the *Megategni*) and Hippocrates's *On Regimen in Acute Diseases*. The Salernitan master, Bartholomaeus of Salerno (fl. ca. 1175), wrote a series of commentaries on the *Articella* and the *Tegni*, which he used as the basis of his teaching. Far from simply reiterating the basic points of the texts, Bartholomaeus sought to use them as a starting point from which he could explore larger theoretical issues in medicine, incorporating Aristotelian and Arabic philosophical learning so as to explain the place of medicine in relation to the larger subject of natural philosophy. As a result, by comparison with the more practically oriented texts previously available in Latin, which focused largely on providing remedies for specific diseases, the new Salernitan medical texts were more concerned with providing theoretical explanations for the underlying causes of disease and justifications for the efficacy of those remedies.

The translations not only encouraged new approaches to medical learning in Salerno but sparked the rise of the first universities across Europe as people sought to assimilate the newly available scholarship on a wide range of subjects, including medicine. Several centers gained a reputation as informal sites of learning in the twelfth century, but over time some developed into a more formalized academic community and institution of instruction known as a *studium generale* or university, which received the right to design curriculum and rules for conferring degrees. By the beginning of the thirteenth century, Salerno had been eclipsed as a center for medical learning by university medical schools, the greatest being the universities in Montpellier, Paris, Bologna, and Padua. Other universities had medical faculties, but they were often small and they had very few medical students, finding it difficult to compete with the larger medical schools. Universities drew students from all over Europe, brought together by the common language of instruction, Latin. Jews, however, were excluded from earning degrees, although in some universities, like Montpellier, they could attend lectures if they paid the appropriate fees. Women were denied access to university education entirely.

The curriculum was remarkably similar in the many university medical schools across Europe. Students would first study the seven liberal arts, which were divided into the *trivium* (grammar, logic, and rhetoric) and the *quadrivium* (arithmetic, geometry, astronomy, and music) in order to receive a bachelor's degree. In addition to these subjects, students would also learn about the natural sciences, based on the works of Aristotle. Following these preliminary studies, a student could opt to pursue an advanced degree in one of the liberal arts, or in one of the higher disciplines of theology, law (canon/ecclesiastical law or civil law), or medicine. The medical doctorate, which conferred the *licencia ubique docendi* (license to teach in any university), required at least ten years of study and was very expensive, so many students would instead pursue a bachelor of medicine degree, conferring the

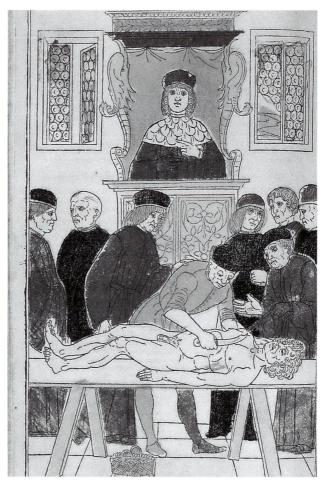

This image is from the title page of the *Fasciculo di medicina*, by Johannes de Ketham (1493). It depicts an anatomy lecture in which a medical student (seated in the high chair) would read from a copy of a learned text on anatomy, while a surgeon would perform the less exalted task of dissecting the body. The professor of medicine (the elderly gentleman to the right with the stick for pointing) would offer additional comments and explanations to expand upon the details described in the text. Students (in their long academic gowns) gather around the body to hear the lecture and discuss the lesson. (Oxford Science Archive/StockphotoPro)

right to practice, which still required several years of study beyond work in the liberal arts.

Following the example set in the *Isagoge* and the *Pantegni*, the medical curriculum was divided into the areas of *theoria* (theory) and *practica* (practice.) Under *theoria*, students would study the philosophy of medicine, physiology (including anatomy), and principles of pathology to understand the causes of disease. Courses on *practica* covered the methods of diagnosis and treatment. Lectures were based upon specific books, most often the books of the *Articella*, and selections from Avicenna's *Canon*, supplemented by short works by Galen and other Greek and Arabic medical authors. University professors would read passages from the selected texts and then provide commentaries and explanations on the passage, typically with reference to other books on medicine. The method of teaching by commentary was reflected in the most popular learned genre of medical writing from this period, the "commentary" on a specific text. Although providing a commentary on a single text might seem reductive, in practice it allowed the lecturer to show his wide knowledge of the written medical tradition as he considered particular *questiones* (questions), or issues under theoretical dispute (e.g., "Can a child raised only by mutes learn to talk?" "Should purgation be done only with drugs in cases of leprosy?," "Is it appropriate to use phlebotomy in cases of strong pain?," or "Do women emit semen, and if so is it necessary for conception?"), which were of significance for elucidating theoretical problems or for actual practice.

The heavy emphasis in the universities on reading and interpreting the books of the ancient medical authorities in the medical schools was intended to provide students with certain, true knowledge, supported by logical argumentation, as opposed to knowledge gleaned through experience in practice, which was considered anecdotal and prone to misinterpretation by the practitioners. This does not mean that university medical students did not receive any practical training. Indeed, they were often required by university statutes to attend a practicing physician and thus gain some experience at the bedside to supplement their theoretical learning. Nonetheless, the distinguishing mark of a university-trained physician would be his theoretical training and command of the written texts of the Greek and Arabic medical authorities; a student who had received a university medical education could claim to understand the humoral theory of health and disease as explained by the Greek authorities and its implications for therapeutic practice. By contrast with non-university-trained healers, therefore, a university physician would claim that his treatments were supported by rational, theoretical medicine, and not simply by empirical practice.

## The Hierarchy of Medical Practitioners and the Non-Learned Tradition of Medieval Medicine

In Latin, the term *medicus* (doctor) could be used to refer to anyone who practiced medicine or surgery, but with the rise of university medicine the term *physicus* (physician) was increasingly used to distinguish a medical practitioner trained at university (and thus familiar with natural philosophy and the theoretical basis of medicine) from other doctors not trained in the written tradition. Throughout the Middle Ages, the *physicus* remained comparatively rare and most people would receive treatment from a range of different kinds of healers arrayed in a kind of hierarchy of prestige.

Those healers below the level of the *physicus* on the medical hierarchy typically learned their craft through some form of apprenticeship or on the job training. Next, in terms of prestige to the *physicus*, came the skilled *chirurgicus* (surgeon), who performed a wide range of surgical procedures including lancing boils, setting bones, conducting lithotomies (a surgical method for removing bladder stones), or even executing difficult operations to reduce hernias. Like the *physicus*, skilled surgeons were also comparatively rare, so that the majority of healers fell into a range of less prestigious occupations. Barber-surgeons, as their name implies, would provide a shave and a haircut, but they also put their sharp knives to use performing minor dental and surgical procedures, such as pulling teeth or letting blood. Apothecaries collected a wide range of spices and herbs and would mix them to produce healing drugs for a fee. At the very bottom of the medical hierarchy, composing the majority of all medical practitioners, one would find a variety of healers who specialized in one kind of procedure (e.g., treating eye diseases, cutting for bladder stones, or setting bones), sold simple herbal remedies, or offered magical or religious healing. Midwives, who were supposed to focus on the treatment of women and children, would also fall into the bottom rung of the medical hierarchy. Despite the fact that physicians commanded more prestige (and higher fees), patients regularly sought aid from all varieties of healers.

While the learned Latin medical tradition remained primarily under the control of the university-trained physicians, who could read the Latin texts, increasingly some of these medical texts were translated into the vernacular languages of Europe. Vernacular translations of recipe books existed in the thirteenth century, but in the late fourteenth and early fifteenth centuries, an increasing number of theoretical medical texts were translated into vernacular languages making them available to a wider medical audience. Soon it was not uncommon for learned surgeons, apothecaries, and other healers, who would not know Latin, to have access to the tradition of learned medicine written in their own language. Thus the dissemination of Greek and Arabic theoretical medicine continued to a wider range of healer (surgeons, apothecaries, and others), at once signifying the respect given to elite medical science and ensuring its enduring value.

# CHAPTER 3

# Religion and Medicine

Faith systems help to explain humanity's place in the cosmos and offer guidance on how an individual can lead a life in harmony with the universe. From this perspective, illness is a state in which the individual fails to attend to his or her physical, mental, or spiritual well-being and hence falls out of alignment with the universe. Religious explanations often ascribed the onset of illness to the influence of gods or other supernatural forces, inflicted either on a whim or as a punishment for sin. Such beliefs necessitated that any cure attend not only to the physical condition but also to the underlying spiritual cause. Therefore, whereas "medicine" is concerned with health in the more limited sense of physical condition, religion has historically taken a more holistic approach that also considers a patient's mental and spiritual well-being. The overlapping interest between religion and medicine in the preservation and restoration of health explains why healers in traditional societies would be equally likely to offer religious, magical, and naturalistic cures.

## FAITH, MAGIC, AND HEALING IN MESOPOTAMIA AND EGYPT

### Gods and the Causes of Disease

In ancient Mesopotamia and Egypt, numerous gods were associated with healing. The goddess Gula, "the great one," was one of the most important healing gods in Mesopotamia, as was the goddess Ninisina, a fertility goddess who was also described as a midwife. Similarly, in Egypt several gods and goddesses were recognized for their general healing powers (especially Osiris, Isis, and Sekhmet), while others offered more specialized medical care (e.g., Serqet offered protection against scorpion stings and the bites of venomous animals, while Bes and Taweret were known for assisting in pregnancy and childbirth). The sick wrote prayers requesting the aid of these deities or wore protective amulets shaped in their likenesses. Indeed, many clay votive offerings to Gula survive, shaped like sick people clutching their afflicted body parts, or in the shape of dogs, her divine symbol.

The gods were not always beneficent but were also known for their role in causing disease. Both the Mesopotamians and the Egyptians believed diseases could be caused by outside malign influences including gods, demons, ghosts, and other supernatural forces. Egyptian medical texts speak of *aaa*, which appears to be a poisonous substance (sometimes the seminal discharge of an incubus) introduced into the body through magical means, and cures are offered for "driving out the *aaa* of a god or goddess," as well as others that refer to the *aaa* of a dead man or woman. Mesopotamian records also express the belief that disease might arise as a punishment for individual sin or for breaking taboos, although it might not always be clear which sin was being punished, as one prayer makes clear:

> Loosen my disgrace, the guilt of my wickedness; remove my disease; drive away my sickness; a sin I know (or) know not I have committed; on account of a sin of my father (or) my grandfather, a sin of my mother (or) my grandmother, on account of a sin of an elder brother (or) an elder sister, on account of a sin of my family of my kinsfolk (or) of my clan . . . the wrath of god and goddess have pressed upon me. (Sigerist 1951, 445)

Wicked sorcerers or other humans might even use incantations or curses to encourage the gods to inflict disease on their enemies. For example, the Code of Hammurabi, written circa 1750 B.C.E., concludes by warning that should any subsequent ruler destroy these codes he would suffer numerous curses:

> May Ninkarrak [a form of Gula, goddess of healing], the daughter of Anum, my advocate in Ekur, inflict upon him in his body a grievous malady, an evil disease, a serious injury which never heals, whose nature no physician knows, which he cannot allay with bandages, which like a deadly bite cannot be rooted out, and may he continue to lament (the loss of) his vigor until his life comes to an end! (Meek 1969, 180)

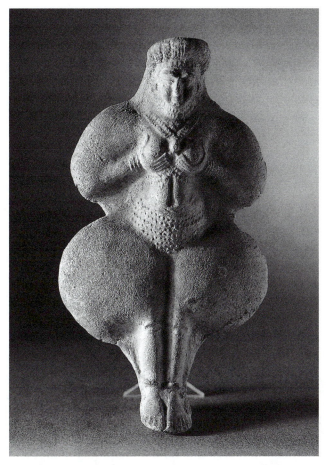

This terracotta Mesopotamian fertility figure (fourteenth–twelfth century B.C.E.), possibly representing the goddess Ninisina, was discovered in what is presently Susa, Iran. Figures like these were kept by women in ancient Mesopotamia to aid in fertility and to offer protection during pregnancy and childbirth. (G. Dagli Orti/De Agostini/Getty Images)

When examining a patient, therefore, the doctor would first need to determine the origin of the condition (i.e., what the patient had done and which being was responsible for the affliction) before being able to determine a course of treatment, which would typically require some form of ritual intervention, to thwart evil incantations or to purify the afflicted in order to placate the gods.

## Religious Healing in Ancient Mesopotamia

Herodotus, a Greek historian writing in the fifth century B.C.E., indicated that the Babylonians in Mesopotamia had no physicians or specialized medical personnel; sick people went to the marketplace where passers-by would offer advice on the nature of the illness and suggest treatment. Although the medical system in Mesopotamia may not have resembled the Greek system that Herodotus knew, it is clear that the Mesopotamians did have an established system of medical treatment and a variety of different kinds of specialists involved in the health care process. One significant difference that may have led to Herodotus's misunderstanding is that in Mesopotamia religion, magic, and science were all united in an inseparable learned system in which naturalistic and religious explanations for diseases coexisted, and cures, whether herbal remedies or charms, were all believed to be imbued with magical or spiritual healing properties. As a result, healers in the Mesopotamian world were typically members of the priestly classes, unlike the *iatroi* Herodotus knew in the Greek world.

Two priestly classes in particular had duties as medical practitioners: the *baru* (diviner) and the *ashipu* (exorcist). Most *baru* appear to have worked directly for the kings, local lords, or the army, thus holding high social status. In addition to their normal duties as diviners, they would be called upon to provide an initial diagnosis of disease by examining omens from the gods and interpreting signs. For example, the *baru* believed that if he should see a black dog or a black pig on his way to the patient's home, then that sick person would die, but if he should see a white pig, then the patient would survive. The *baru* would also examine sheep entrails, in which they believed the gods "wrote" messages, to divine the cause of illness. Numerous handbooks survive that list the various discolorations and markings in the entrails that the *baru* would observe, along with a description of their significance. They also made use of clay models of sheep livers that indicated specific points of interest on the liver and provided brief annotations about their significance to aid in divination. Beyond having a role in making the initial diagnosis to identify the cause of the disease, however, it appears that the *baru* was not involved in treatment.

The *ashipu* was a priest who performed purification rituals or exorcisms to cleanse temples and other spaces in preparation for religious ceremonies. Most of their activities, therefore, had nothing to do with treating illness. They were also adept at interpreting the various omens that could aid in prognosis and diagnosis, however, and unlike the *baru*, the *ashipu* could perform the rituals necessary to purify a sick person by driving out the evil spirits causing the disease and then reconciling her or him with the gods. They also provided patients with various healing incantations. For example, a cure for an eye affliction required that the healer take threads of red and white wool and tie seven knots in each, and then placing the red thread over the injured eye and the white thread over the healthy eye he should recite a charm such as this one: "O clear eye, O doubly clear eye, O eye of clear sight! O painful eye, O doubly painful eye, O eye of painful sight! A pair they are one eye, yet a mountain is set as a bar between them . . . (on) their surface a knot is tied, (on) their under parts a wall is built" (Thompson 1924, 31). The *ashipu* was also capable of offering herbal drugs that could be taken while reciting a healing charm, as with this remedy for the disease caused by "hand of a ghost":

> If a man has been seized by a ghost and the *ashipu* is unable to get it to withdraw, you crush together the following [a list of unidentifiable plants follows], you rub him with oil, you wrap up (the herbal mixture) in a piece of leather and put it around his neck. If "hand of a ghost" is persistent in a man's body and cannot be gotten rid of, to expel it you take (various minerals) and carob seeds, you char them over coals, you pulverize them, you mix with cedar resin; you recite (the following) incantation seven times. (Biggs 2005, 12–15)

In many respects, therefore, the *ashipu* would offer the same kinds of healing services as the *asu* (doctor), indicating that little distinction was made between religious and naturalistic healing in Mesopotamian society.

## Magical Cures in Egypt

There is ample evidence that a variety of magicians and priests, distinct from the *swnw*, practiced medicine in ancient Egypt. Many, like the *sau* magicians, made protective charms and amulets that could be used to protect against disease or during pregnancy. The *wab* priests of Sekhmet, the lion-headed goddess, were also recognized as important healers, although they played a slightly inferior role to the *swnw*. Sekhmet was believed to bring pestilence and famine, and thus her priests played an important role in healing since people needed to appease her to prevent disease. These individuals practiced comfortably alongside the *swnw*, and indeed the *swnw* often also had the title of magician, suggesting that he combined both roles in his own practice.

The *swnw* also regularly incorporated magical healing into his repertoire, and several incantations or spells that can be used for healing are listed alongside herbal remedies in the medical papyri. For example, the Ebers papyrus offers this incantation against *wekhedu*:

I trample Busiris; I throw down Mendes; I ascend to the sky to see what is done therein. Nothing will be done in Abydos until the driving out of the [evil] influence of a god, a goddess, male *wekhedu*, female *wekhedut*, and so on, and the influence and all evil things that are in this my body, in this my flesh and in these my limbs. . . . I will not say: I will not repeat: Perish as you came into being! Words to be said four times and spat out over the site of the disease. Really effective: a million times. (Nunn 1996, 105)

Therefore, as was the case in Mesopotamia, Egyptian healers were prepared to offer a combination of religious, magical, and naturalistic cures.

## RELIGIOUS AND NATURALISTIC MEDICINE IN ANCIENT GREECE

Homer's *Iliad* (written during the eighth century B.C.E.) describes the god Apollo spreading plague among the Achaeans encamped before the walls of Troy by firing disease arrows at them until "the corpse-fires burned on, night and day, no end in sight. Nine days the arrows of god swept through the army" (Fagles 1990, 79). In response, the Achaeans consulted a soothsayer to determine how they had offended Apollo and what they would need to do to propitiate him and end the plague. Following the soothsayer's advice, they purified themselves and made appropriate sacrifices to placate Apollo, and only then did the plague cease.

The gods were also known for curing disease, and Greek patients who sought religious healing could invoke a wide range of gods, including Apollo who was the leading healing deity in the Greek pantheon. Increasingly from the third century B.C.E. onward Asclepius, who was recognized for his healing abilities in Homer's *Iliad*, eclipsed Apollo as the primary healing god, and his cult spread throughout the Mediterranean region. In early myths, Asclepius was said to be the mortal son of Apollo and a mortal mother, known for his knowledge of drugs and incantations for use in healing, but over time he came to be recognized as a god in his own right and the Greeks built several temples dedicated to him. Sick people could travel to one of his temples and undergo purification rites before being allowed to enter the *abaton*, or sacred dormitory, where they would sleep for the night. They believed that Asclepius would appear in their dreams and either cure them or offer advice on how they could procure a treatment. After recovery, many supplicants left inscriptions thanking the god for his divine cure, like the one left by Ambrosia of Athens, who had been blind in one eye:

She came as a suppliant to the god. As she walked about in the Temple she laughed at some of the cures as incredible and impossible, that the lame and the blind should be healed by merely seeing a dream. In her sleep she had a vision. It seemed to her that the god stood by her and said that he would cure her, but that in payment he would ask her to dedicate to the Temple a silver pig as memorial of her ignorance. After saying this, he cut the diseased eyeball and poured in some drug. When day came she walked out sound. (Edelstein and Edelstein 1998, 230)

In another inscription we learn that Asclepius revealed this remedy to a man who had suffered a cough for two years: "Italian wine flavored with pepper to drink; then again starch with hot water, then powder of holy ashes and some holy water, then an egg and pineresin, then again moist pitch, then iris with honey, then a quince and a wild purslane to be boiled together" (Edelstein and Edelstein 1998, 252). The prescription, which mixes holy substances with more ordinary ingredients, suggests that religious and naturalistic healing continued to comfortably coexist in the Greek world. By the end of the first century B.C.E., the cult of Asclepius was so widespread that, of all the pagan gods, he was the only serious competitor to Christ as a healing god.

By contrast to the evidence from the Homeric period and the religious healing offered in the temples to Asclepius, the Hippocratic authors in the fifth and fourth centuries B.C.E. sought to provide naturalistic explanations for disease and hence naturalistic cures. The most obvious expression of this idea is found in *On the Sacred Disease*, which discusses the condition of epilepsy. The early Greeks believed that this disease was caused by divine visitation—hence the name "sacred disease"—and the cure consisted of undergoing a process of ritual purification and reciting healing incantations. The author of *On the Sacred Disease*, however, vigorously counters the perception that the "sacred disease" is caused by the gods, declaring that charlatans and faith healers invoke a divine cause for the ailment merely to account for their failure to cure it. Rather, he explains the disease within the naturalistic framework of the nascent humoral theories, declaring that epilepsy is caused by excess phlegm on the brain, and offers a number of empirical proofs and anatomical explanations for the disease. As to the cure, the author declares,

This disease styled "sacred" comes from the same causes as others, from the things that come to and go from the body, from cold, sun, and from the changing restlessness of winds. . . . Whoever knows how to cause in men by regimen moist or dry, hot or cold, he can cure this disease also, if

he distinguish the seasons for useful treatment, without having recourse
to purifications and magic. (Jones 1923, 183)

The Hippocratic authors did not necessarily deny the value of religious cures, but they did seek to separate naturalistic and religious
healing and to mark the *iatros* as one who offered natural, not magical
or religious, remedies for disease.

## MEDICINE AND RELIGION IN INDIA AND CHINA

### Magic and Medicine in Early Indian and Chinese Civilizations

The earliest medical beliefs in India and China bear a strong resemblance to those of ancient Mesopotamia and Egypt. The four sacred
scriptures of the Hindu religion that were written during the Vedic
period in India (ca. 1500–500 B.C.E.), the *Rigveda*, the *Yajurveda*, the
*Samaveda*, and the *Atharvaveda*, described the religious rituals to be
performed by the Brahmans, or priestly class. One of these texts, the
*Atharvaveda*, is less concerned with the rituals of sacrifice and prayer
and more focused on materialistic and naturalistic matters, containing a number of magical incantations aimed at providing protection
against demons, witchcraft, and natural disasters. It describes a number of illnesses caused by demons, poisoning, or accidents, and reveals
several incantations and magical charms aimed at protecting against
those diseases, and also for ensuring fertility and a successful pregnancy, promoting hair growth, or generally guaranteeing a long life. In
this tradition, the *bhishaj*, professionals who combined the craft medical
knowledge of artisans with the intellectual learning of priests, would
be expected to know the appropriate incantations and spells to cure
specific ailments and also how to produce amulets and talismans from
plants and other substances that could ward off demons and malign
spells in order to bring about a cure. In its earliest origins, therefore,
Vedic medicine was based in a system of healing magic and Ayurvedic
medicine was profoundly shaped by this tradition.

During roughly the same period in China, in the time of the Zhou
dynasty (1045–256 B.C.E.), disease was also conceived of as having
divine or supernatural causes. Chinese demonic medicine was based
on the belief that demons or other evil spirits would inflict illness on
individuals. The earliest surviving Chinese medical texts, discovered
in the Mawangdui gravesites, which date to about 168 B.C.E., including the *Wu-shih-erh ping fang* (*Fifty-Two Prescriptions against Fifty-Two
Ailments*), reveals a belief in the demonic cause of disease and provides a variety of magical spells and talismans to ward them off. The

*wu,* shaman-like practitioners who offered the curing incantations and talismans, would also sometimes use herbs and other medicinal substances as remedies to treat demon-related illnesses. These beliefs bear a striking resemblance to the magical medicine of the Vedic period in India.

### Confucianism and Taoism in Chinese Medical Thought

The life of Confucius (551–479 B.C.E.) and the spread of Confucian philosophy coincided with the political and social chaos of the late Zhou dynasty and Warring States (ca. 475–221 B.C.E.) periods. Confucian thought was oriented around the question of how to organize social life in order to maintain political harmony and end warfare. As it gained adherents, Confucianism also influenced the early development of traditional Chinese medicine, in particular offering a metaphorical way of thinking of the body as a well-ordered state, as can be seen in the *Huangdi Neijing* (*The Yellow Emperor's Classic of Internal Medicine*):

> The heart is the sovereign of all organs and represents the consciousness of one's being. It is responsible for intelligence, wisdom, and spiritual transformation. The lung is the advisor. It helps the heart in regulating the body's *qi.* The liver is like the general, courageous and smart. The gallbladder is like a judge for its power of discernment. The pericardium is like the court jester who makes the king laugh, bringing forth joy. The stomach and spleen are like warehouses where one stores all the food and essences. . . . [So the] *zang* and *fu* organs must work together harmoniously, just like a kingdom. . . . It is in this way that one's life is preserved and perpetuated, just as a country becomes prosperous when all its people are fulfilling their duties. If the spirit is disturbed and unclear, the other organs will not function properly. This creates damage. The pathways and roads along which the *qi* flows will become blocked and health will suffer. The citizens of the kingdom will also suffer. These are the relationships of a kingdom. (Ni 1995, 34)

In this way, the maintenance of health required that the individual regulate all aspects of his life and body, just as a king would manage a peaceful and ordered state. By extension, disease was envisioned metaphorically as political or social breakdown that would disrupt the flow of communication and commerce.

The teachings of Taoism, founded by the philosopher Lao-Tzu (sixth century B.C.E.), also spread in China in response to the political and social disruption during the Warring States period and had a similar influence on the direction of traditional Chinese medicine. Whereas

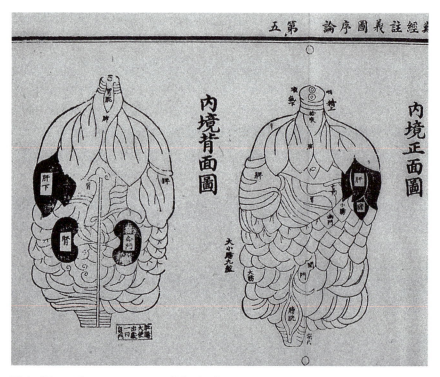

This fifteenth-century woodblock illustration is based on a medical text from the Song dynasty in China. It depicts the internal organs of the body from the front (*left*) and back (*right*). (Wellcome Library, London)

Confucianism emphasized the goal of creating political and social order among humans, Taoism was more concerned with teaching how man should conform to "the Way" and live in harmony with nature. For some, the pursuit of harmony with nature was equated with the pursuit of longevity. The *Huangdi Neijing* refers to the "Perfect Ones" of antiquity who had achieved these goals:

> In the past, people practiced the Tao, the Way of Life. They understood the principle of balance, of *yin* and *yang*, as represented by the transformation of the energies of the universe. Thus, they formulated practices such as Dao-in, an exercise combining stretching, massaging, and breathing to promote energy flow, and meditation to help maintain and harmonize themselves with the universe. They ate a balanced diet at regular times, arose and retired at regular hours, avoided overstressing their bodies and minds, and refrained from overindulgence of all kinds. They maintained well-being of body and mind; thus, it is not surprising that they lived over one hundred years. (Ni 1995, 1)

As is evident in this passage, Taoism envisioned a holistic approach to health that emphasized exercise, meditation, and diet as a means to maintain health. Although Taoism did not deny the role of demons in causing disease or the use of magic as cures, its emphasis on nature encouraged naturalistic explanations for illness and the continued development of pharmacological knowledge and herb lore as another means of curing disease.

In this way, the early writings in traditional Chinese medicine are founded upon diverse systems of belief. Confucianism and Taoism together offered a philosophical structure for the early development of medical theories. Both systems drew upon the cosmological theory of systematic correspondence, the theory of *yin* and *yang*, and the doctrine of *wu xing* ("five phases"). They offered a philosophical framework within which to understand the functioning of the human body as it related to society and the wider cosmos, which overlay the earlier beliefs of demonic medicine. Furthermore, they also emphasized a system of health care that defined health as more than simply physical well-being, but more broadly as the state of harmonious balance between body, soul, society, and the cosmos.

## Buddhism in Indian Medicine

From the fourth century B.C.E. onward, Buddhist ascetics (monks and nuns), who gathered in monastic communities called *sanghas*, took on the role of healing the sick within their community and sometimes even traveled to heal others in the surrounding areas. Many of these monks pursued knowledge about medical theory and practice, learning the medical beliefs of the *bhishaj*, and they played a significant role in collecting, editing, and writing down the content of the oral tradition of magico-religious Vedic medicine.

At the same time, however, they were also greatly influenced by the empirical medical learning passed on by ascetic wanderers from North India called *sramanas*. The *sramanas* were generally known for their empirical and rational approach to disease and treatment, placing less emphasis on magical healing than the Vedic tradition. Unlike the Brahman healers, they held no taboos about touching dead bodies and encouraged ascetics to learn anatomy by dissecting animals and observing decomposing human bodies. Furthermore, the early sramanic texts offer more naturalistic herbal remedies and medicinal foods as cures, with less emphasis on magical cures than in Vedic medicine. As a result, the early Ayurvedic texts that were finally written down by Buddhist monks (including the *Caraka* and the *Susruta*) unite the empirical and rational approaches of the *sramanas* with the magico-religious healing of the Hindu Vedic tradition (Zysk 1998).

The Buddha was frequently referred to as the "king of physicians" for his emphasis on helping the suffering. Indeed, his spiritual contemplation began with witnessing disease, old age, and death in the natural world, and he taught that healers should consider the eightfold causes of disease: an imbalance in one of the three *doshas*, changes of the seasons, engaging in unusual or excessive activities (sitting or standing too long), emotional stresses (being assaulted by a robber or arrested as an adulterer), or the result of previous actions (karma). The recognition of the theory of the three *doshas* and other naturalistic and physical causes of disease (seasons and excessive activity) reaffirms the rational approach to healing present in the Buddhist tradition that influenced Ayurvedic medicine. However, the Buddha's classification of disease placed equal emphasis on the physical, mental, and spiritual causes of suffering. Mental suffering, which typically arose from the emotions of greed, anger, or ignorance, required that patients seek a cure through meditation and spiritual contemplation. Nonmonastic Buddhist texts also reflect a comingling with indigenous magico-religious healing traditions. For example, in Tibetan Buddhist medicine magical healing became an integral part of the ascetic's healing arsenal; they would offer protective charms, rituals, and mantras that could ward off supernatural causes of disease and purify the individual to reverse the effects of karma. As Buddhism spread, the more magico-religious form of Buddhist medicine as well as the empirico-rational monastic medicine explicated in the *Ayurveda* were both exported to neighboring countries in Central Asia.

## FAITH HEALING IN THE ISLAMIC AND CHRISTIAN TRADITIONS

### Prophetic Medicine in the Islamic World

With the spread of Islam from the seventh century onward, Muslim scholars compiled treatises purporting to reveal the "Medicine of the Prophet" as an alternative form of healing for pious Muslims, who opposed the Greek medical philosophy, which often made use of medicinal substances that were forbidden by Islamic law. These texts included collections of quotations on sickness and therapeutics drawn from the Quran and the hadith, sayings attributed to the Prophet Muhammad (d. 632). Specific conditions, including fevers, leprosy, plague, nosebleeds, and headaches are all addressed in the Prophetic Medicine manuals, as are other more esoteric calamities such as the "Evil Eye," a condition that some authors felt the need to defend as real.

The treatment provided in the Prophetic Medicine treatises was generally fairly minimal. Surgery was barely mentioned, aside from circumcision. Cautery, bloodletting, cupping, the regulation of diet and regimen, and the use of drugs formed the core of the naturalistic treatments offered. Simple drugs were favored over compound medicines, honey being perhaps the most commonly prescribed medicinal substance. In addition, these treatises present several prayers and incantations that could be used in aid of a cure. One such incantation was offered in a cure for treating colic:

> Write for him [the patient] the opening surah of the Quran, the surah "Purity," and the two surahs for seeking protection [the last two surahs of the Quran, "Dawn" and "People"]. Then write underneath: "I take refuge in the presence of God, the Great, and in His might, which is unceasing, and in His power, which nothing can resist, from the evil of this pain, and the evil within it." Then swallow with rainwater on an empty stomach. You will be cured of it, God the exalted permitting. (Pormann and Savage-Smith 2007, 150)

The emphasis here is on the belief that God will provide a cure. Talismans and amulets were also often used to ward off epidemics and other diseases or to alleviate the suffering of women during a difficult childbirth.

Although several physicians trained in Greek humoral medicine questioned the efficacy of using amulets, talismans, and other magico-religious healing techniques, there was often considerable overlap between these two healing systems. Some Prophetic Medicine manuals drew upon the medical learning available in texts based on the Greek tradition and even sought to reconcile the two traditions, emphasizing that although God would provide the cure for disease, humans still needed to discover it and apply it correctly. At the same time, physicians were not always ready to rule out the efficacy of magical or occult cures. Some even included various amulets and other magical cures alongside herbal remedies in their medical texts; one physician recommends placing a lock of hair from a dead person on a painful tooth to alleviate the pain, or placing the hair under the head of a sleeping person to help him sleep longer. In this way, Prophetic Medicine managed to coexist with the philosophical Greek medical tradition in the Islamic world.

## Magical and Miracle Cures in Medieval European Medicine

In the ancient world, Christianity was widely recognized as a healing religion. Christ was regularly described by the early church fathers as *Christus medicus* (Christ the doctor) and as a result, Christianity competed for followers with other religions devoted to healing gods, like the cult of Asclepius. The New Testament describes a number of miracle cures provided by Jesus, and evidence throughout the course of the fourth century C.E. suggests that Christians increasingly attested to witnessing miraculous healing and sought divine aid to restore health. This does not mean that Christians eschewed secular medicine or that they did not visit physicians trained in the Greek tradition. In the eleventh century C.E., Bishop Fulbert of Chartres described the relations between religious and secular healing in a hymn:

> As Christians we know that there are two kinds of medicine, one of earthly things, the other of heavenly things. They differ in both origin and efficacy. Through long experience, earthly doctors learn the powers of herbs and the like, which alter the condition of human bodies. But there has never been a doctor so experienced in this art that he has not found some illnesses difficult to cure and others absolutely incurable. . . . The author of heavenly medicine, however, is Christ, who could heal the sick with a command and raise the dead from the grave. (Park 1992, 64)

Fulbert's account indicates that he saw the two healing systems as complementary, but noted the limitation of secular medicine in the case of certain intractable conditions in comparison to the extraordinary possibilities of heavenly medicine.

People seeking miracle cures in the Middle Ages would typically turn to the cult of saints. Supplicants could pray to a particular saint, or in many cases go on a pilgrimage to visit the shrines of saints where they could receive a miraculous cure by touching the saints' relics, drinking the waters in which they had been dipped, or sleeping near the saint's tomb. Monks associated with the shrines kept records of the miracle cures performed by their saints, like these:

> A man crippled from birth got about by dragging himself along with hand-trestles. His thumb, too, was bent back, the nail nearly through the palm. While huddled at Godric's tomb crying and moaning he straightened his legs and began to extend them. During this many heard a crackling noise of bones and ligaments stretching. At dawn he arose and walked up to present the trestles as an offering; his hand was healed, only a red spot remaining in the palm.

Matilda, a young girl, felt a swelling and pain in her right breast and then there was a discharge from nine openings in the afflicted part. After human medicines failed, she vowed some wax to William of Norwich and applied it to her breast; relief followed when she removed the wax. She went to the cathedral to offer the wax, and baring her breast applied it to the tomb, after which the disorder was completely cured. (Finucane 1977, 91, 105)

The monks' lists of cures offer insight into the variety of conditions for which people sought divine healing. Among adults, the most common cures were for cripples and paralytics, followed by cures for the deaf, mute and blind, then cures for the mad or possessed. Other conditions receiving miracle cures included wounds, sterility, tumors, and various skin conditions (such as leprosy). This list suggests that most supplicants sought heavenly healing for chronic conditions that were not otherwise susceptible to treatment by secular medicine and in general they undertook the expensive pilgrimage to a shrine only after the doctors had failed to bring about a cure.

Although all saints might be called upon for miracle cures, certain saints were renowned for curing specific diseases. Saint Sebastian and Saint Roch were associated with the plague, for example, while Saint Lazarus was associated with leprosy, Saint Agatha with breast cancer, Saint Mathurin with mental illnesses, and Saint Maur with gout. In an unusual case in southern France, some people venerated a greyhound (known for its loyal service protecting a child) as a "saint" and they brought their sick children to the shrine of "Saint Guinefort" for healing. On the other hand, other saints were recognized for their more general healing abilities, including Saint Job (renowned for being afflicted with a number of diseases) and Saints Cosmas and Damian (brothers who had been physicians in life and were recognized as the patron saints of doctors). The sick could offer intercessory prayers requesting heavenly healing to any of these saints, in lieu of going on an actual pilgrimage; in many cases, they might promise to go on a pilgrimage to the shrine of the saint after the cure had been performed.

Starting in the twelfth and thirteenth centuries, physicians trained in the Greek humoral tradition in the universities began to grow increasingly skeptical of magical and religious folk medicine. Nonetheless, many scholastics continued to include magical cures using amulets and charms in their medical writings for a number of reasons. Sometimes physicians cynically suggested that they only included magico-religious cures to provide patients with what they expected or because they thought these cures could still have a positive psychological effect on patients. Other physicians argued that even though they could not provide rational explanations for the efficacy of magical incantations and amulets, they might still function according to some unknown occult property—just as they could not explain the power of the magnet to attract iron shavings, for example. Magico-religious elements appear frequently in certain circumstances in scholastic texts, such as when discussing treatments for conditions for which rational remedies seemed ineffective. For example, the physician Valesco de Tarenta (fl. 1382–1418) attested to his own successful use of certain religious charms to treat epilepsy, which he says should be recited three times into the patient's ear: "Jesus of Nazareth, crucified king of the Jews" or "Gaspar brings myrrh, Melchior frankincense, Balthazar gold." Furthermore, he claims that the patient should have these phrases written on a clean sheet of paper and suspended from his or her neck to ward off future epileptic fits. In similar fashion, the learned surgeon Teodorico Borgognoni (d. 1298) reported a ritual and incantation for use when extracting arrows from wounds:

> It does not trouble me to write down at the end of this chapter certain empirical experiments, although they have not been tested by me, experiments which I know certain experienced men swear by.
>
> Therefore, for the purpose of drawing out an arrow, let there be said thrice, on bended knee, The Lord's Prayer (that is, the paternoster), and when these have been said, let the arrow be grasped with both hands joined as they are, and let be said, "Nicodemus drew out the nails from our Lord's hands and feet, and let this arrow be drawn out," and it will come out forthwith. (McVaugh 2003, 320)

Teodorico may not have been fully convinced of the efficacy of this ritual, noting that he had not tried it himself, but he still felt the need to include it in his list of treatments for a condition that frequently proved fatal.

# CHAPTER 4

# Women's Health

The single greatest cause of death among women in the premodern world was complications attending childbirth, and premodern societies often recognized that women were prone to different diseases from men and thus required differentiated care. The field of gynecology encompassed not only the treatment of "women's diseases" but almost every aspect of female health care, and it is linked to the field of obstetrics, which focuses on the care of women during pregnancy and childbirth. In premodern societies, the care of women often fell to midwives, especially in the context of managing pregnancies and childbirth, but that was not always the case; male practitioners wrote extensively about how to treat "women's diseases" and also on how to manage complications during birth, and they likely treated female patients in many of these circumstances. In this chapter, we will examine the ways in which women's health care was understood, methods of treating women and managing the birthing process, and the range of practitioners involved in treating female patients.

## GYNECOLOGY: WOMEN'S BODIES AND WOMEN'S DISEASES

### Mesopotamia and Egypt

It is not clear which practitioners were most involved in providing women's health care in ancient Mesopotamia and Egypt. Midwives, called *sabsutu*, assisted in childbirth in Mesopotamia, but evidence indicates that *asu* and *ashipu* were also called in to treat women and attend to complications following childbirth. In ancient Egypt, there are no known words for midwife, gynecologist, or obstetrician, but there is no documentary evidence to indicate that the *swnw* was specifically involved in childbirth, although it is clear they were called on to treat women patients. This raises a question about the extent to which the male practitioners who produced the written medical texts were actually involved in treating women or knew about female anatomy.

Mesopotamian healers did not understand or write extensively about female reproductive anatomy or diseases specific to women. By contrast, several Egyptian medical texts survive that discuss women's health, and the Kahun papyrus is devoted specifically to the subject of gynecology. The Kahun papyrus attributes women's illnesses mainly to the activities of the uterus. This is true not only of what we might consider uterine diseases; for example, a woman whose eyes are aching until she cannot see or one with aching in her molars or ears is diagnosed as having discharges or terrors of the womb. Different medicinal remedies were prescribed for these conditions brought on by the uterus, often including fumigating the uterus with incense or other substances like burning goose fat or dried human excrement. Egyptian texts also offer many remedies for "cooling the uterus" and "driving out heat," or this one: "Instructions for a woman suffering in her vagina, and all her limbs likewise, having been beaten. You shall say concerning her: 'This has loosened her uterus.' You should then prepare for her: oil to be eaten until she is well" (Nunn 1996, 197). These descriptions of women's illnesses and their cures imply that the *swnw* typically viewed all aspects of women's health as being specifically related to the uterus.

Fertility was probably the major concern reflected in Mesopotamian and Egyptian gynecological literature. The Kahun papyrus and other Egyptian medical texts offer a number of tests to determine whether a woman was even fertile like this one: "[To determine] who will [bear children] and who will not [bear children], you should then cause the bulb of an onion to spend the night in her flesh until dawn. If the odor appears in her mouth, she will bear [children]. If [it does not], she will never [bear children]" (Nunn 1996, 192). Likewise, in both medical traditions we find medical prescriptions and magical incantations aimed at helping women conceive or curing sterility. One Mesopotamian prescription for making a barren woman conceive reads, "Total: twenty-one stones to help a barren woman become pregnant; you string them on a linen thread and put them around her neck" (Biggs 2005, 9). The main emphasis of gynecological medicine, therefore, appears to have been to ensure that a woman be able to conceive and bear children.

## Greek and Roman Gynecological Literature

The Hippocratic corpus includes several treatises that consider female physiology and gynecology, including *Diseases of Women*. These texts explain women's health in terms of the regularity or irregularity of menstruation or in terms of the motions of the uterus. Accordingly, retention of the menses, excessive menstruation, and "suffocation" of the womb were considered significant illnesses and therapies (including diet, regimen, and drugs) were provided to alleviate the uterus and restore the proper flow of the menses. Furthermore, according to the Hippocratic *On Generation*, "if [women] have intercourse with men their health is better than if they do not . . . Intercourse by heating the blood and rendering it more fluid gives an easier passage to the menses; whereas if the menses do not flow, women's bodies become prone to sickness" (Lonie 1981, 4). Likewise, in *Diseases of Women I*, the author addresses the importance of intercourse for maintaining women's health and also describes numerous afflictions of the womb:

> If suffocation [of the womb] occurs suddenly, it will happen especially to women who do not have intercourse and to older women rather than to young ones, for their wombs are lighter. It usually occurs because of the following: when a woman is empty and works harder than in her previous experience, her womb, becoming heated from the hard work, turns because it is empty and light. There is, in fact, empty space for it to turn in because the belly is empty. Now when the womb turns, it hits the liver and they go together and strike against the abdomen—for the womb rushes and goes upward toward the moisture, because it has been unduly heated by hard work, and the liver is, after all, moist. When the womb hits the liver, it produces sudden suffocation as it occupies the breathing passages around the belly. . . . When the womb is near the liver and the abdomen and when it is suffocating, the woman turns up the whites of her eyes and becomes chilled; some women become livid. She grinds her teeth and saliva flows out of her mouth. . . . If the womb lingers near the liver and the abdomen, the woman dies of the suffocation. (Hanson 1975, 576)

These diseases of women reflect a societal expectation that women should be engaged in reproduction for the sake of their own health— failure to engage in intercourse and thus maintain regular menstruation and placate the womb could be fatal.

Greek physicians and natural philosophers also considered the physiological differences between male and female bodies, and these discussions often revolved around beliefs about their respective contributions to conception. In his work *Generation of Animals*, Aristotle (384–322 B.C.E.) described female bodies in relation to the humoral and qualitative theories, arguing that female bodies were colder than male bodies. As a result, he maintained, their bodies were unable to produce a fully formed seed and thus they only contributed a lesser, material substance to conception that did not influence the child's physical form. On the other hand, he believed that male bodies, due to their heat, could produce a fully active seed, which impressed itself on the material substance produced by women's bodies to provide the form or blueprint for the future child. Later, Galen of Pergamum (129–ca. 216 C.E.) challenged Aristotle's one-seed theory, claiming that both male and female bodies contributed a seed to conception and in partial proof of this he pointed to the fact that offspring often resembled their mothers. These competing theories from the two preeminent medical and biological scholars of antiquity about the differences between male and female bodies would have significant influences on later understandings of sex difference and reproduction in European medicine.

## Gynecology in Ayurvedic Medical Literature

As in the Greek world, the *Susruta Samhita* and the *Caraka Samhita* both view menstrual irregularities as the main source of women's diseases. The *Susruta* indicates that menstruation begins at age twelve and ceases at age fifty with the onset of the perceptive deterioration of the body. During those years, the regulation of the menses is deemed crucial because it is the essential factor that makes impregnation possible, along with male semen. Irregular menstruation was usually attributed to derangement of the *doshas* and treated by diet and drugs, when necessary.

Medical and religious texts offer extensive advice to aid with impregnation. Foremost, they recommend a regimen to be followed after the start of the menses: for the first three days the woman should remain chaste, but after taking a cleansing bath on the fourth day the following nine days are deemed most suitable for conception. If conception occurs on even days after the onset of the menses (fourth, sixth, eighth, tenth, or twelfth day) she will have a boy, if on odd days (fifth, seventh, ninth, eleventh) she will have a girl. The *Susruta* also indicates that conception under unusual circumstances might present a danger to the future offspring:

A boneless (i.e., with cartilaginous bones) monstrosity is the outcome of the sexual act in which both the parties are female and their Súkra (sexual secretion) unite somehow or other in the womb of one of them. Fecundation may take place in the womb of a woman, dreaming of sexual intercourse in the night of her menstrual ablution. The local *vata* carries the dislodged ovum into the uterus and exhibits symptoms of pregnancy, which develop month after month till the full period of gestation. The offspring of such a conception is a Kalah (a thin boneless jelly-like mass) on account of the absence of the paternal elements in its development. Such monstrosities as serpents, scorpions, or gourd shaped fetuses delivered from the womb of a woman should be ascribed as the effects of deadly sins. (Bhishagratna 1911, 132)

Sterility and other problems hindering conception are explained as being caused by derangement of the *doshas* that lead to the production of impure sperm or menstrual blood. Therefore, the Ayurvedic texts offer a number of tests to determine the potency of sperm and menstrual blood; for example, incurable impotency can be diagnosed if the sperm or menstrual blood smells like urine or feces. A variety of remedies are otherwise offered to cure impotence, including dietary changes, sweating, and drugs—women are prescribed pastes applied as vaginal suppositories.

## Gynecology in Traditional Chinese Medicine

The *Huangdi Neiching* (*The Yellow Emperor's Classic of Internal Medicine*) envisioned male and female bodies in terms of a balance of yin and yang but did not attend extensively to anatomical differences. Indeed, the uterus played virtually no role in early Chinese medical writings— the *zang* and *fu* organs were the main anatomical structures present in both male and female bodies and the uterus received little attention except in brief discussions of pregnancy. Reproductive powers were associated with the kidneys (a *zang* organ) for both sexes and they were deemed responsible for fertility and conception. In this learned medical system, male and female bodies were thought to be prone to the same diseases and were treated similarly. In popular practice, however, evidence suggests that women's health care was the domain of a range of female healers (*nü yi*), herbalists, acupuncturists, masseuses, and shamans, suggesting that women did indeed receive differentiated medical treatment.

Sun Simiao (581–682 C.E.) was the first medical author to emphasize the medical importance of sexual difference, arguing that, "the disorders of women are ten times more difficult to cure than those of males," and "for women, there are separate prescriptions [from those appropriate for men]" (Furth 1999, 26, 51). Following Sun Simiao's lead, the field of *fuke* (translated as gynecology) arose, examining the range of diseases and therapies of "wives" (a *fu* is a married woman), and it developed into a mature specialization during the Song dynasty (960–1279 B.C.E.). Gradually, *fuke* became an academic subject and was taught in the state-approved schools of the Imperial Medical Bureau, where learned male physicians sought to establish their own authority to provide for women's health care, especially in the imperial palaces. In 1220, a professor of medicine celebrated the development and spread of *fuke* as a medical specialty:

> For the first time there is specialized knowledge concerning the women's chambers. Surely it should not fail to be written in books? I have made a study of this specialization in medicine. Not daring to be lazy and disregarding my own ignorance, I have gathered many prescriptions and compiled them into a volume called *One Hundred Questions on Medicine for Females*. (Furth 1999, 69)

His book was intended as a kind of bedside manual for family use, not directed specifically at learned physicians, indicating that by his time the field of *fuke* was gaining popular recognition beyond court practice.

With the rise of the specialty of *fuke*, menstruation received greater attention in medical diagnosis, as a visible marker of female reproductive functioning, often earning the most extensive coverage in gynecological sections of medical texts. One Song physician, Chen Ziming (ca. 1190–1270 C.E.), maintained, "In treating illness in women, one must first regulate the menses, so I place this first." Furthermore, he advised physicians, "In males one regulates *qi*, in females one regulates Blood [since] . . . in women Blood [function] is the root" (Furth 1999, 75). Following this theory, treatises on *fuke* recognized three broad categories of women's diseases: wind stroke (*zhongfeng*), depletion fatigue (*xusun, xulao*), and swellings and accumulations (*jiju*). All of these presumed a deep-rooted pathological disorder of the blood and *qi* in women that could disrupt the menses or impair sexual and reproductive function. For this reason, *fuke* manuals prescribed drugs for women that were known for their ability to "enliven Blood," "replenish Blood," or "move Blood." One of the most popular, the "Four Ingredients" infusion (*Siwu tang*), contained angelica root and white peony root (both known for their blood-nourishing properties), lovage rhizome (believed to improve the proper movement of blood), and fresh rehmannia root (believed to move *qi* in the body).

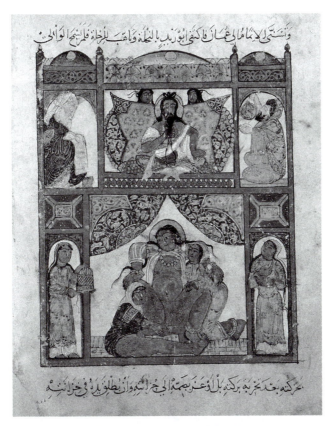

This thirteenth-century Persian illustration depicts a queen giving birth with the aid of female attendants. Male physicians were not typically present during childbirth. (Bibliotheque Nationale, Paris, France/Archives Charmet/The Bridgeman Art Library)

## Female Practitioners and Women Patients in the Islamic World

Women healers played an important role in Islamic society and they did not only treat women patients. Learned physicians often bemoaned the extent to which patients felt free to turn to these women healers:

> How amazing it is [that patients are cured at all], considering that they hand over their lives to senile old women! For most people, at the onset of illness, use as their physicians either their wives, mothers or aunts, or some [other] member of their family or one of their neighbors. He [the patient] acquiesces to whatever extravagant measure she might order, consumes whatever she prepares for him, and listens to what she says and obeys her commands more than he obeys the physician. He believes that this woman, despite her lack of intelligence, is more knowledgeable and of sounder opinion than the physician. (Pormann and Savage-Smith 2007, 103)

Learned male physicians, however, were aware that female patients were often unwilling to seek medical care from men, especially for women's conditions. In these cases, it is most likely that women continued to seek the care of female healers.

Male physicians in the Islamic tradition did write extensively on topics relating to gynecology and obstetrics, even if they mostly repeated material found in their Greek sources. Furthermore, it is clear that male physicians were sometimes consulted to treat female patients. Al-Razi (d. ca. 925, known as Rhazes in the Latin West), for example, reports treating a woman with a breast tumor and al-Zahrawi

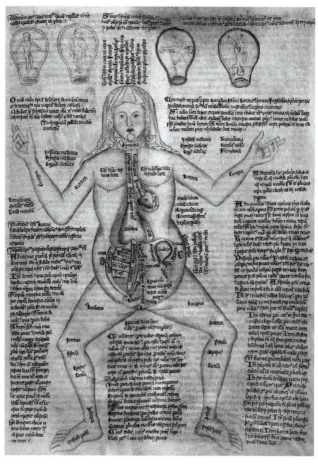

This image of "disease woman" was produced in a Latin text around 1420–1430. The names of various diseases are marked on the parts of the body they affect. Across the top, four images show a fetus in utero, depicting different kinds of fetal presentations one might encounter during birth. (Wellcome Library, London)

(fl. ca. 1000, known as Albucasis in the Latin West) reports treating a girl with a knife wound in her throat and two other women with growths on their head and neck. Al-Zahrawi even describes the surgical use of forceps to perform a surgical operation on a woman to extract two fetuses that had died in utero. Despite these accounts, however, it appears that the practice of gynecology and obstetrics in the Islamic world remained in the hands of women practitioners.

## The "Secrets of Women" and Male Physicians in Medieval Europe

One influential thirteenth-century text in Europe, the *De secretis mulierum* (*On the Secrets of Women*), erroneously attributed to the Aristotelian natural philosopher Albertus Magnus, purports to reveal the secret knowledge women have about their bodies that gives them control over human reproduction. Many physicians wrote commentaries on this text, expanding on the ideas it contained, and it was even translated into several vernacular languages, attesting to the popularity of the text among both learned medical men and the literate lay public. The text covers a wide range of sexual, gynecological, and obstetrical topics and elaborates on the power women have to promote or prevent conception, influence the sex of the fetus in utero, procure abortions, and otherwise act against the interests of men seeking male heirs. Furthermore, some passages portray women as sexually avaricious and wicked, warning that, "when men have sexual intercourse with these women it sometimes happens that they suffer a large wound and a serious infection of the penis because of iron that has been placed in the vagina, for some women or harlots are instructed in this and other ill deeds" (Lemay 1992, 88). Menstruating women are described as especially dangerous and one later commentator expanded upon this point:

> When men go near these [menstruating] women they are made hoarse, so that they cannot speak well. This is because the venomous humors from the woman's body infect the air by her breath, and the infected air travels to the man's vocal cords and arteries causing him to become hoarse. It is harmful for men to have sexual intercourse with menstruating women because should conception take place the fetus would be leprous. This also frequently causes cancer in the male member. (Lemay 1992, 130)

Writing in French, Christine de Pizan (1363–ca. 1430), the daughter of a physician at the French royal court, strongly denounced the *De secretis mulierum* for its disparaging portrayal of women. However, in the paternalistic medieval society concerned with producing male heirs, the popularity of this text reflected a general misogynistic fear of the power women had over the reproductive process.

Concurrently with the rising popularity of the *De secretis mulierum* in the fourteenth and fifteenth centuries, learned university physicians started to write a number of original texts on gynecology and obstetrics. Many of these texts are written with the stated intention of providing better theoretical gynecological knowledge and training for midwives. However, these books also reflect the male physicians' efforts to establish their own authority to treat all aspects of women's health and to supervise, if not entirely supplant, midwives in these activities. Indeed, their writings suggest that physicians were increasingly active in the treatment of women. One physician, for example, writes about his own experience in applying a rotten hen's egg to cure a woman's prolapsed uterus, boasting, "I marveled at its immediate reduction," and then indicating that he tried it on another woman with similar success (Green 2008, 252). Accounts of male physicians having gained such intimate access to female patients are rare, however; medieval physicians continually lamented the fact that women were reluctant to seek their advice for menstrual disorders until the condition was so advanced that it was difficult to treat.

## OBSTETRICS: MANAGING PREGNANCY AND CHILDBIRTH

### Childbirth in Ancient Mesopotamia and Egypt

Although medical texts from ancient Mesopotamia offer numerous prescriptions to treat women with difficulties during pregnancy, parturition, and complications after childbirth, care during the delivery of babies mostly rested in the hands of the *sabsutu*, midwife, who was likely assisted by female relatives and other women. Prior to birth, the *asu* and *ashipu* were concerned with dangers associated with profuse vaginal bleeding, which they feared would lead to miscarriage, and offered a number of medicinal substances (applied as potions, tampons, vaginal fumigations, or salves) used in concert with magical charms to alleviate the bleeding. Mesopotamian healers believed that profuse bleeding leading to miscarriage could be caused by sorcery or evil magic. Therefore, many of the incantations were designed to prevent the evil spells from taking effect:

> If [you want] sorcery not to approach a pregnant woman, [and] for her
> not to have a miscarriage, you crush magnetite, antimony, dust, subu-

stone and dried "fox" grape. You mix [the resulting paste] with the blood of a female shelduck and you take [it] with cypress oil and you rub [it] on her heart, her hypogastric region and her [vulva's] "head" and you tie on a band [made from] a cloth [made] of red-colored wool (or you take a potsherd [found] standing on edge at a crossroads and you bury it in the inner threshold and sorcery will be kept at bay) and you put masculine su-stone on her left hand. (Scurlock 1991, 135–183)

In this case the use of the red-colored wool likely had magical symbolism associated with blood and the potsherd buried behind the door likely symbolized the intention to ward off intruders from outside. These protective medicines and incantations would have been provided by the *asu* and *ashipu* who knew such rituals and indicates that they did have a role in caring for pregnant women.

It is possible that some women may have wanted to procure an abortion. One Mesopotamian text provides a prescription "to cause a pregnant woman to 'drop' her fetus," listing eight ingredients that should be mixed in wine and given to the woman to drink on an empty stomach and ends with the words, "that woman will 'drop' her fetus" (Biggs 2005, 9). Unlike the evil magic of sorcerers aimed at causing an unwilling miscarriage in women, this drug appears to have been designed for use at the woman's request, but it is not clear how it would have been used. Although this drug could have been used to hasten delivery or to expel a dead fetus, it is also possible that it may have been administered to provoke an abortion. Assyrian law codes specifically demanded the death penalty for women who self-aborted, however, suggesting that the use of such a drug with the specific intention of provoking an abortion would have carried severe risks. The vague way in which the results of the prescription are described may, in fact, reflect this supposition.

The *sabsutu* was expected to perform many rituals in the birthing chamber designed to protect the mother from the dangers of childbirth. For example, for a woman with an overly narrow birth canal the *sabsutu* could recite this incantation: "The woman in travail is having difficulty giving birth; she is having difficulty giving birth. The infant is stuck fast; the infant is stuck so fast as to end (her) life. The door bolt is secure; the door is made fast against the suckling kid" (Scurlock 1991, 141). She could also apply numerous lubricants in conjunction with massaging the abdomen to help hasten the labor. The lubricants were often composed of substances having magical symbolism such as hailstones, dust from fallen walls, or dust from leaky drainpipes as one text describes: "Like a hailstone (which can never go back to the heavens), may the (fetus) not be able to return to what is behind him.

Like one who has fallen from a wall, may he not be able to turn his breast. Like a leaky drainpipe (which cannot hold water), may none of the (mother's) waters remain" (Scurlock 1991, 141). Difficulties during birth could have natural causes, but medical texts also presumed the possibility that evil sorcerers were at work. Such threats would likely have required the use of more powerful incantations that are found in the medical texts, suggesting that the *asu* and *ashipu* probably stood ready to provide assistance as necessary during difficult births.

Although there are no known words for midwife or obstetrician from ancient Egypt, it is likely that women were the ones assisting during childbirth as in other ancient cultures. No documentary

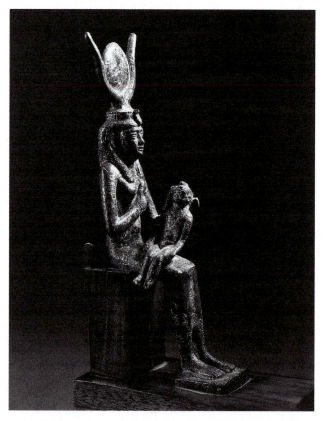

This statue represents the Egyptian goddess Isis nursing her child, Horus. Isis protected Horus from snakes and other predators when he was an infant, and for this reason she was viewed as the ideal mother and was also believed to protect mortal children from harm. Statues like this one could be kept to provide protection to mothers and children. (G. Dagli Orti/De Agostini/Getty Images)

evidence indicates the involvement of the *swnw*, but medical texts do offer advice for managing birth. Medical papyri described tests to determine whether a woman was pregnant or determine the sex of the fetus in utero. Mothers wanting a male child would often drink milk from a woman who had recently delivered an infant boy, and mother's milk was sometimes stored in special jars shaped like a mother nursing her baby for such use. Medical texts also included prescriptions that could be used as contraceptives: "Beginning of the prescription prepared for women/wives to allow a woman to cease conceiving for one year, two years or three years: *qaa* part of acacia, carob, dates; grind with one *henu* of honey, lint is moistened with it and placed in her flesh [i.e., in her vagina]" (Nunn 1996, 196). Other recipes for contraceptives recommend the application of crocodile excrement! Finally, there are also several remedies and some incantations for hastening birth and for helping to expel the placenta. Based on these sources it is clear that the *swnw* was interested in the birthing process, but the descriptions are often vague, suggesting that he would not customarily take part in the delivery.

## Childbirth in Ancient Greece and Rome

In ancient Sparta, childbirth was depicted as a glorious act; the Spartans only allowed the names of warriors who died in battle and women who died in childbirth to be inscribed on their tombstones! In other parts of the Greek and Roman world, however, women giving birth were not depicted in such glowing terms. In addition to being dangerous, childbirth was also viewed as being polluting for the mother and child in the ancient Greek and Roman world. Indeed, rules associated with sacred districts stipulated that people could not die and women could not give birth in the precinct for fear of polluting the holy area. As a result, mothers and newborns were regarded as vulnerable immediately after birth and were kept secluded for a period before being reintroduced into the general household after undergoing necessary purification rituals.

Midwives were the ones primarily involved in attending to the needs of pregnant women and assisting in the delivery of babies. Soranus of Ephesus (fl. 100 C.E.) describes the midwife's responsibilities and the birthing process in his work on gynecology and obstetrics. The midwife, he says, was responsible for making certain that the necessary oils, lubricants, sponges, and warm water for cleaning were available, as well as bandages, swaddling, and a pillow for the newborn after birth. She would oversee the woman in labor, providing necessary drugs and comforts to assist until it was time to deliver, at which point the woman would move to a special birthing stool, with a crescent-shaped opening in the bottom and solid crossbars for handles that she could grasp during contractions. The midwife would then be ready to advise the woman on breathing, while directing her assistants and preparing to receive the infant when it appeared. According to Soranus, this was a difficult job and he listed a number of stringent requirements for any woman who would undertake it: she should be literate (presumably so as to read his book!), physically strong with delicate fingers and short finger nails, able to remain calm under pressure, and be of good moral character. Soranus's text implies that learned doctors would be ready to step in and assist in cases of difficult births, but even then they would have needed to work in concert with the midwife to bring about a safe delivery. He describes in great detail how the midwife would widen the birth canal if necessary and how she should turn the fetus in the womb in cases of difficult presentations. Above all, he advises that she remain calm, "for we see many alive who have thus been born with difficulty" (Temkin 1956, 189). It seems that Soranus clearly intended to imply that he knew more about delivering babies than the midwives!

Soranus expected that midwives would step aside and call in physicians in cases where it was necessary to extract a dead fetus from the uterus, yet another dangerous complication of childbirth, and he describes the tools and procedures for performing this operation. Although popular stories maintain that Julius Caesar was born through a "caesarean" section, giving his name to the procedure, it is unlikely that a true C-section was performed in the Greek or Roman world. As proscribed by Roman law, such procedures were only performed on women who died during childbirth, with the intention of saving the child; this was a measure of last resort and it was not performed on live women to save the mother's life in cases of difficult births. As Caesar's mother is said to have survived to give birth to other children and to learn of his invasion of Britain, she clearly had not undergone such an operation.

The Greeks and Romans did describe a number of drugs that could be used as contraceptives or to promote abortions. The Hippocratic *Oath* specifically forbids a doctor to provide an abortive suppository to women, but the author of a different Hippocratic text, *On the Nature of the Child*, recommends the "Lacedaemonian leap" in which the woman would leap in the air and kick her heels to her buttocks to expel the seed from her womb, implying that other methods of abortion or contraception were possibly acceptable. Other Hippocratic texts describe recipes for a variety of contraceptive medicines. Soranus, recognizing the discrepancy in these Hippocratic texts sought to distinguish between abortive and contraceptive measures, indicating that the Lacedaemonian leap could be interpreted both ways, and he makes clear the fact that these methods could be controversial in his own day:

> [One] party prescribes abortives, but with discrimination, that is, they do not prescribe them when a person wishes to destroy the embryo because of adultery or out of consideration for youthful beauty; but only to prevent subsequent danger in parturition if the uterus is small and not capable of accommodating the complete development, or if the uterus at its orifice has knobby swellings and fissures, or if some similar difficulty is involved. And they say the same about contraceptives as well, and we too agree with them. And since it is safer to prevent conception from taking place than to destroy the fetus, we shall now first discourse upon such prevention. For it is much more advantageous not to conceive than to destroy the embryo. (Temkin 1956, 63)

Nonetheless, after describing various methods for preventing conception, Soranus also gives detailed advice on how to provoke an abortion—recommending a number of herbal drugs, violent exercise, leaping vigorously, and being shaken around by riding in carriages. Indeed, his apprehension about abortion revolves more around a fear that the drugs could be harmful to the woman than a specific opposition to the goal of provoking a miscarriage. Similarly, many later Greek and Roman texts included recipes for both contraceptives and abortifacient, like this one from the second century C.E.:

> Take 1 drachma iris, 1 drachma Cnidian grain, 1 drachma galbanum, 1 drachma turpentine. Mix in equal parts with lily oil, Cyrian oil (consisting of omphacine oil [Lesbian wine], sweet flag, myrrh, *aspalathus*, cardamom, and flowers of Cyperus Rose oil). . . . Insert into the vagina before a bath with fenugreek and Artemisia. If this does not produce an abortion, let her repeat the procedure but this time inserting the suppository after the bath with these: wallflower (or stock) seed, soda, and wormwood soaked in wine on wool pad. (Riddle 1992, 95–96, 100)

Other evidence suggests the widespread availability of amulets and charms for the same ends. Thus, although some physicians as well as several legal and literary texts from this period expressed opposition to abortion, it appears that many people made use of such methods.

## Childbirth in India

Childbirth was not generally handled by physicians in India, but rather by midwives. Nonetheless, Ayurvedic medical texts offer substantial advice on the care and observation of pregnant women. Indeed, the *Susruta* emphasizes that the care of the pregnant woman had dire consequences for fetal development:

> The child of a mother whose wishes are not honored and gratified during pregnancy stands in danger of being born palmless, hunchbacked, lame, dumb or nasal voiced through the deranged condition of the *vata* of its mother's body. The malformation of a child in the womb should be ascribed to the atheism of its parents, or to the effects of their misdeeds in a prior existence, or to the aggravated condition of the *vata, pitta,* and *kapha.* (Bhishagratna 1911, 132–133)

Thus, the pregnant woman was supposed to avoid physical labor, sexual activity, sleeping during the day, staying up late at night, and being frightened; rather, she should spend her time in pleasant surroundings, eat good food, and be carried around in a carriage whenever she needed to travel. Advice is also given for recognizing whether a pregnant woman was carrying a male, female, hermaphrodite child, or twins, based on the shape of her belly, development of breasts, facial features, and posture. The sex of the fetus was also thought to dictate the woman's desires (e.g., food preferences) and needs during pregnancy, hence these signs could also be observed to determine the sex of the offspring.

The medical texts also consider cases of difficult labor (*mudhagarbha*) in which the fetus presents in the wrong position leading to an obstructed delivery. Various texts describe a number of abnormal fetal presentations (e.g., the fetus descends with both legs first, with one arm stretched forward, etc.) and indicate that these complications are dangerous and could lead to fetal death. Facing these situations, the midwife's assistants were supposed to recite appropriate mantras while she introduced her hand anointed with ghee (clarified butter) into the vagina and repositioned the fetus. The *Susruta* describes two fetal presentations that should be given up as hopeless since the obstructions cannot be corrected. A fetus in these positions is called *viskambha* ("bolt"), and the text indicates that it will need to be surgically removed. The procedures and tools required for this operation are described in detail. The *Susruta* expects that a male surgeon will perform the operation, although another text indicates that the procedure would be entrusted to a clever midwife. In any case, the mother's survival was probably fairly unlikely and the texts recognize this, even requiring that the surgeon receive the ruler's permission before starting the operation.

In the event that the mother should die during labor, the *Susruta* provides directions for performing a caesarean section: "A child, moving in the womb of a dead mother, who had just expired (from convulsions, etc.) during parturition at term, like a goat should be removed immediately by the surgeon from the womb as a delay in extracting the child may lead to its death" (Bhishagratna 1911, 58). The indication here is that the surgeon would need to take over in this case and it implies that the procedure was readily known since it was practiced on animals—possibly why the *Susruta* does not offer any other details of the operation. The earliest recorded case of a caesarean section in India is that of Bindusara (ca. 320–272 B.C.E.), the second Mauryan emperor, whose mother accidentally consumed poison and died when she was about to deliver, necessitating that he be cut from her womb.

Abortion and miscarriage are discussed in the Ayurvedic texts. The medical understanding of embryological development explained that in the first four months the fetus is in a liquid state so any termination of the pregnancy would be called an abortion; in the fifth and sixth months the limbs begin to solidify so after this point it is called a miscarriage. The texts suggest that an abortion could be triggered by many causes, including insufficient food, food that is especially heavy, warm, or pungent (particularly intoxicating beverages), excessive physical exercise, sexual intercourse, suppression of natural excretions, dire emotions (especially anger and fear), and emetic or purgative drugs. Although the medical texts do not explicitly suggest that women might seek to have an abortion, the recognition that certain drugs could provoke an abortion indicates that the possibility of using them in this way existed. Child abandonment was practiced in India, as in other ancient cultures, thus other methods of regulating family size were also available.

## Childbirth in China

*Chanke* (obstetrics) rose to prominence as a medical specialty in China during the Song dynasty, at the same time as the field of *fuke* (gynecology) was developing. Previous works like Zan Yin's (fl. 852–856 C.E.) *Chanbao* (*Treasure of Childbirth*) had indicated increasing medical interest in the subject of childbirth, but it was not until the Song period that it was widely recognized as a distinct medical subdiscipline within the field of *fuke*, of interest to learned male medical practitioners. Previously, childbirth had been the realm of women healers, the *nü yi*, who did not have access to learned theories on pharmacy or acupuncture. Indeed, popular stories from earlier centuries suggest that physicians were only called in at the last minute to assist with complications arising during childbirth, and their intervention consisted of prescribing drugs and performing acupuncture.

Chen Ziming's *Furen Daquan Liangfang* (*All-Inclusive Good Prescriptions for Women*) was the best-known text from the Song period on obstetrics. Rejecting what he saw as the spiritualism of Buddhist books

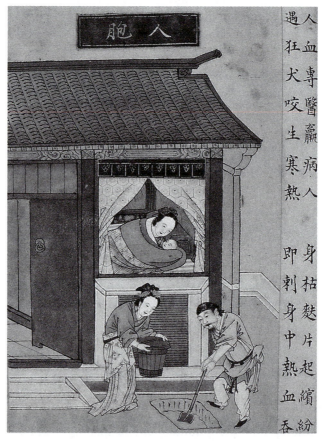

This sixteenth-century Chinese illustration is titled *Human Placenta*. It depicts a mother and her newborn resting in their home, shortly after delivery. Meanwhile, in the foreground a man digs a hole to receive the placenta, which is carried out by another woman in a chamber pot. According to Chinese tradition, the placenta was buried in order to assure the mother's and newborn's health. (Wellcome Library, London)

and *wu* shamans and the superstitions of old women, Chen Ziming endorsed the natural philosophical model of gestation, envisioning the "ten months of pregnancy," that conformed to the theory of the Five Phases and thus understood the significance of pregnancy within the context of the Chinese zodiac and the greater cosmos. He believed that armed with this knowledge and, by implication the guidance of physicians, pregnant women would be able to know how to ward off the ghostly fetuses and "wandering fetus killers" that threatened the health of the pregnant woman and her fetus. Furthermore, Chen Ziming's advice gave instructions on how to consult the special birth charts (*chan tu*), which would dictate information such as the preparation of the birthing chamber (e.g., the placement of the birthing couch, the curtains, and even the door) and also where the placenta should be buried after delivery to ensure the mother's and child's health. In this way, his work aimed to direct the ritual practices associated with childbirth in accordance with rational natural philosophy and medical theory.

Song physicians also increasingly wrote about intervening in cases of difficult childbirth. Again, Chen Ziming played a leading role, transmitting and augmenting an older text on different kinds of abnormal deliveries in his own medical work. He presents himself as offering advice for the women who would be assisting during delivery, noting, "Few delivery women have subtle and clever hands, and for this reason many [pregnant women] are endangered. Because I grieve for their plight, I must offer assistance" (Furth 1999, 121). While he emphasizes his own authority on the subject of *chanke* (especially in cases of difficult labor and delivery), it is clear that Chen Ziming did not attend to women in childbirth on his own. Rather, he intended his text as an instruction manual for women who would handle the process of childbirth, implying that he would work in concert with them to bring about a successful delivery. Learned male physicians may have been exerting their authority to enter the birthing chamber during this period, but they had not taken it over entirely.

One interesting story from the twelfth century C.E. gives some insight into Chinese attitudes toward abortion:

There was a woman in the capital named Bai; she was beautiful and the city people all called her Peony White. She sold abortifacients for a living. All of a sudden she was afflicted with brain sickness. [Her head] daily swelled larger and none of the famous doctors of the city could cure her. By day it suppurated and stank unbearably, and nightly the neighbors heard her groans. One day she called her household together and said, "You are to burn my entire collection of abortion prescriptions; I warn you, my children and disciples—you cannot carry on this calling." The sons said to their mother, "Our mother has made the family livelihood from this. How can we throw it away?" The mother said, "Every night in my dreams hundreds of infants gnaw at my skull, making me cry out in pain. This is all retribution because I used poisonous drugs to ruin fetuses." Having spoken thus, she died. (Furth 1999, 123)

Bai's final decision suggests that the use of abortifacients could be seen as immoral, leading her to worry that her own illness was brought on by the fetuses aborted by her medicines—indeed, the ghosts of aborted and miscarried fetuses were believed to pose a threat to pregnant women. On the other hand, her family recognized that selling abortifacients was a lucrative business—many people were buying medicines from the lady called "Peony White" (white peony was a known abortifacient). Chen Ziming offered prescriptions to make "nuns, prostitutes, or ailing wives" barren or to "cut off birth" in cases in which the pregnant woman's health was endangered, showing that physicians were also aware of such medicines (Furth 1999, 168). However, physicians were concerned about the dangers of provoking abortions and warned that care should be taken when doing so. Thus, despite laws prohibiting infanticide and abortion in China, the medical stance and story about Bai suggest that abortifacients were commonly available to those who sought them.

## Childbirth in Medieval Europe

The birthing chamber continued to be almost exclusively under the control of women during the Middle Ages. Men (male relatives, priests, physicians, surgeons) were only infrequently present in the birth chamber. As a result it seems that this space stirred much fascination, engendering numerous stories from the period about the escapades of men who dressed up as women in order to infiltrate this feminine world and discover its secrets (although court records indicate that these men were often sneaking into birth chambers in order to find eligible women companions). Male physicians also tried to assert their authority to enter this feminine realm. Over the course of the fourteenth and fifteenth centuries C.E. physicians increasingly wrote about the need to instruct and supervise midwives. For example, in addition to his Latin texts on the subject, Michele Savonarola (1385–1468) wrote a manual in Italian, the *Regimen for the Women of Ferrara*, with the explicit aim of instructing midwives and other women in the city of Ferrara on matters of obstetrics. Although male physicians and surgeons probably did not wish to displace midwives in most cases of obstetrical care, their texts imply that they were skilled in handling a variety of obstetrical difficulties, especially those that might require surgical intervention.

The management of difficult labors and obstetrical surgery received extensive coverage in Latin medical texts. The performance of caesarean sections to extract a living fetus from a woman's womb after she had died received particular attention. Theologians and priests emphasized the benefits of this operation since it would allow the child to be baptized, ensuring its eternal survival, even if there was little expectation that the child would survive long after the baptism. Furthermore, medical authors described a number of different methods for performing this operation, suggesting that male medical practitioners (physicians and surgeons) were increasingly performing or at least supervising such procedures. The texts also describe methods for dismembering a dead fetus so that it could be extracted surgically to save the life of the woman, thereby emphasizing their expertise in surgical care during obstetrical emergencies.

Contraception and abortion were controversial subjects, especially as far as priests and theologians were concerned in the Middle Ages. General consensus, however, seems to have been that women knew how to prevent conception or procure abortions whenever they chose. Regarding abortion, the popular *De secretis mulierum* (*On the Secrets of Women*), which existed in numerous vernacular translations, reported that excessive physical exertion on the part of pregnant women could provoke the menses and cause a miscarriage. The author follows this observation in typical misogynistic fashion, impugning the morality of women:

> For this reason harlots, and women learned in the art of midwifery, engage in a good deal of activity when they are pregnant. They move from place to place, from town to town: they lead dances and take part in many other evil deeds. Even more frequently they have a great deal of sex, and they wrestle with men. They do all these things so that they might be freed from their pregnancy by the excessive motion. The reason for their great desire for coitus is that the pleasure that they experience will help them blot out the grief that they feel from the destruction of the fetus. (Lemay 1992, 102)

However, many medical authors were less worried about the morality of sexual activities. While acknowledging the religious and moral mandates against sexual intercourse and various practices that might encourage nonreproductive sexual activities, many physicians still felt free to describe recipes for contraceptive medicines and different drugs and methods that could be used to "provoke the menses," which in many cases may have been intended to produce an abortion in pregnant women. Nonetheless, even if physicians chose not to pass on their knowledge about contraceptives and abortifacients, evidence suggests that they were indeed available and well known in the Middle Ages.

# CHAPTER 5

# Health in Infancy, Childhood, and Old Age

## AGING AND THE LIFE CYCLE IN PREMODERN MEDICAL THEORIES

Infant and child mortality rates were high in premodern societies; some estimates suggest that 30 to 40 percent of children died before the age of five, most of those before age one. If a person survived childhood, he could achieve an old age, but average life expectancy was still low. As might be expected, given the high infant and child mortality rates and lower life expectancies, far greater attention is given in the medical texts to considering the health care needs of infants and children, but physicians did also consider some conditions of old age and the treatment of the elderly. In many cases, children and the elderly were viewed as similarly weakened and thus in need of similar medical accommodations, for example, in terms of the dosage of drugs provided.

The Ayurvedic tradition recognizes a correlation between the *doshas* and age, noting that *vata* (wind) predominates in old age, *pitta* (bile) in middle age, and *kapha* (phlegm) in childhood. Childhood lasts to age sixteen and is characterized by rapid growth; in adulthood vitality achieves its high point, lasting to age fifty-five after which old age ensues with a period of mental and physical deterioration. The *Susruta Samhita* advises physicians to tailor all drugs according to the age of the patient so that "the use of strong or drastic purgatives, and cauterization are alike prohibited in cases of children and old men. They should be used only in weakened or modified forms if found indispensably necessary" (Bhishagratna 1907, 323). This recommendation reflects the general concern that the young and the old face different medical concerns and require different forms of treatment.

In traditional Chinese medicine, the aging process is attributed to the waning of yin in the body, so that by age forty the yin is reduced to half its natural capacity and vitality starts to degenerate. According to the *Huangdi Neiching*, "At the age of fifty the body grows heavy and the ears no longer hear well nor is the vision of the eyes clear any longer. At the age of sixty the life-producing force of *yin* declines and impotence sets in." Furthermore, reflecting its Taoist influences and the importance of following "the Way" to achieve a healthy harmony in life, it maintains that those who achieve the appropriate balance in their lives can prevent the depletion of yin and thus "will retain good hearing and clear vision, their bodies will remain light and strong, and although they grow old in years they will remain able-bodied and flourishing" (Veith 1972, 121).

The Western medical tradition, guided by the theory of the relationship among the four humors and four qualities in the body, reflects similar notions about the life cycle and aging to those seen in Ayurvedic and Chinese medicine. Aristotle (384–322 B.C.E.) had observed that the innate heat of a body gradually diminishes the body's moisture over its lifespan, and Galen of Pergamum (129–ca. 216) later expanded upon this idea to identify the innate heat as the primary quality necessary for life. In the thirteenth century in Europe, a number of scholastic physicians took up this notion and further developed it to consider how an individual's complexion or personal humoral balance would change throughout life and lead to a natural death. In brief, these theories maintained that nutrition was necessary not only for growth but also to repair parts of the body consumed by the innate heat. The *humidum radicale*, otherwise known as the "radical" or "seminal" moisture, was deemed the other fuel necessary for maintaining the body's innate heat. Although the exact nature and abundance of this substance was the subject of much theoretical debate, in general the radical moisture was thought to be the most fundamental fluid, which derived from the seminal seed involved in reproduction and as such carried the formative virtue of the soul. Thus, once the body was unable to assimilate nutrition properly and/or had been drained of the vital *humidum radicale*, the body's innate heat would run out of "fuel" and be extinguished, resulting in a natural death. Defined in this way, aging is viewed as a process of drying out characterized by the youthful age of intense heat and activity, followed by a gradual decline in middle age, and then the drying out (and shriveling up) associated with old age. At each stage of life, therefore, people's complexions would change, making them susceptible to different diseases as well as necessitating different forms of therapeutic intervention.

## PEDIATRIC MEDICINE

### Mesopotamian Cures for Children

The Mesopotamians feared that children, newborns in particular, were in danger of assault by demons that would result in disease. Many different medical practitioners had roles in protecting infants and children from such dangers. From the beginning, midwives were expected to perform protective rituals on newborns soon after delivery. A midwife would cut the umbilical cord with a special knife or sliver of reed, wash the infant, and apply oils to its chest while reciting special incantations. After these protective rituals had been performed the infant would be presented with objects appropriate for its sex: weapons for a boy, a spindle or other domestic items for a girl. After the initial protective rituals performed by the midwife, the *asu* (physician) might be asked to treat sick children with his incantations and herbal medicines, but in most cases the care of infant illnesses seems to largely fall to the *ashipu* (exorcist), who specialized in performing the necessary rituals to expel invading demons.

One ancient Mesopotamian tablet was devoted entirely to the medical problems of infants, and others also had specific cures for treating the diseases of children. A number of specific demons were believed to threaten the lives of infants and were associated with particular conditions; the most widely recognized being the Kubu-demon, lilu-demons (and their female counterparts, lilitu-demons), and the most fearsome demoness, Lamastu. Kubu-demons were ghoulish beings that especially directed their malevolence against newborns. References to Kubu-demons as ones who were "not buried in a grave" or as "little ones who do not know their own names (and) who never saw the sun" suggest that they were conceived of as demonic manifestations of stillborn children. They were commonly believed to cause harm to newborns: "If it [the infant] cries during the evening without interruption and does not want to drink milk, it is the hand of Kubu. If (the infant) wheezes before it is put to bed, it is the hand of Kubu. If it continually cries and wheezes, it is the hand of Kubu" (Scurlock 1991, 135–185). In order to dispel these demons, parents would provide personal names for stillborn children in an attempt to make them feel welcome in the family and thus less inclined to inflict harm on their live sibling. Furthermore, it appears that midwives worked a protective ritual on the afterbirth, symbolic of a stillborn twin to the newborn, to turn its attention away from the baby, which had been separated from it when the umbilical cord was cut.

Lilu-demons and lilitu-demons were the ghosts of young men and women who had died before they had the opportunity to marry or have children themselves. They were supposed to sneak into people's homes seeking other children to become the husbands or wives they never had. The *ashipu* could perform a ritual to unite lilu-demons and lilitu-demons in marriage and send them to a properly provisioned home in the underworld, thus placating them and turning their attention away from snatching living children.

The most frightening threat to infants and children was the demoness Lamastu, a minor divinity and daughter of the sky-god Anu. Lamastu is often described as a hideous woman seeking to steal children to nurse as her own. No wonder that the symptoms she causes are sometimes associated with nursing: "If the infant is continually frightened at its mother's breast (and) cries continually, or if it is continually disturbed (and) he jumps from the lap of his mother and cries a lot, the daughter of Anu has chosen him" (Scurlock 1991, 155). Furthermore, she was associated with fevers, abdominal distension, cramps, diarrhea, dizziness, and convulsions in children. The *ashipu* would make offerings to Lamastu in order to induce her to turn her attentions away from the sick child or to fulfill her need to be a mother. One elaborate cure directed at Lamastu requires the *ashipu* to speak an incantation and perform a ritual:

> [Speak the incantation] "I have married you to a black dog, your slave; I have poured out well water for you, (so) let up, go away, withdraw and distance yourself from this little one, child of his god." . . . [The ritual to go with the incantation]: (On the first day in the morning), you make a Lamastu represented as imprisoned. You arrange offerings; you put twelve breads made from unsifted flour before her. You pour out well water for her. You marry her to a black dog. For three days you have her sit at the head of the patient. You put the heart of a piglet in her mouth. You pour out hot broth for her. You put out dried bread for her. You give (her) a wooden *sikkatu*-vessel full of oil. You provide her with (provisions). You recite the spell (every day) in the morning, noon, and evening. On the third day in the late afternoon you take her out and bury (her) in the corner of a wall. (Scurlock 1991, 157)

Many dedicatory plaques made for Lamastu show her riding in a boat filled with her various presents and accompanied by a dog and a piglet, which she is suckling. Interpreted in relation to the plaques, the ritual appears as a kind of bribe and an effort to get her to turn her maternal attentions toward the piglet.

The selection of wet nurses posed another significant consideration for parents seeking to maintain their infant's health. Indeed, the use of wet nurses was prevalent enough in Mesopotamian society to merit attention in the Code of Hammurabi (ca. 1750 B.C.E.): "When a seignior gave his son to a wet-nurse and that son has died in the care of the wet-nurse, if the wet-nurse has then made a contract for another son without the knowledge of his father and mother, they shall prove it against her and they shall cut off her breast because she made a contract for another son without the knowledge of his father and mother" (Meek 1969, 175). Given the health dangers associated with nursing, parents would want to be certain that the nurse did not take on other children, possibly reducing the care and feeding their own child would receive.

## Egyptian Cures for Children

Like the Mesopotamians, the ancient Egyptians employed a variety of religious and magical cures to protect infants and children. One example:

> Mayest thou flow away, she who comes in the darkness and enters in furtively, with her nose behind her, and her face turned backwards, failing in that for which she came!
>
> Hast thou come to kiss this child? I will not let thee kiss him! Hast thou come to silence (him)? I will not let thee set silence over him! Hast thou come to injure him? I will not let thee injure him! Hast thou come to take him away? I will not let thee take him away from me!
>
> I have made his magical protection against thee out of clover (that is what sets an obstacle), out of onions (what injures thee), out of honey (sweet for men, but bitter for those who are yonder), out of the roe of the *abdju*-fish, out of the jawbone of the *meret*-fish, and out of the backbone of the perch. (Wilson 1969, 328)

The Egyptian medical papyri also reflect the importance of religious and magical rituals designed for the care of infants and children. In the Ebers papyrus, we find a number of tests to assess the viability of the infant immediately after birth: if the baby cries *ny* (yes) it will live, but if it cries *mebi* (no) it will die; or, if when turned head downward it groans, it will die. The Ebers papyrus does not specify what to do in response to these tests, but in the Ramesseum IV papyrus, which is devoted to problems of childbirth and neonatal care, a different test is proposed: the *swnw* is advised to give a piece of the placenta rubbed in milk to the newborn and if it is vomited the child will not survive. This test is followed by recommendations for protective incantations and rituals that should be performed for the child on the day it is born. Magico-religious cures are not uncommon in the medical papyri, but the high proportion of them among cures for infants suggests just how tenuous early life was.

Medical papyri also offer more naturalistic cures and treatments for children. They explain common procedures like the ligation of the umbilical cord in some detail and discuss alternative methods for giving drugs to newborns, who cannot swallow pills—the medicine could be rubbed with fresh milk on the mother's nipples prior to nursing, or the mother could take it directly, suggesting the belief that its curative powers would be passed on to the child through her milk. Certain drugs are prescribed for infants to induce them to accept the breast, another remedy prescribes a medicine including poppy to stop children from crying, and sucking on a fried mouse was recommended for children with teething pains. Different remedies (combining drugs and incantations) are offered for the medical conditions of older children, such as retention of the urine, cough, the *baa* disease (characterized by fatigue of the heart, green lips, and weak knees), as well as to stop bed-wetting.

The ancient Egyptians also performed circumcisions on some young male children. The Greek author Herodotus reports that the Egyptians were the first people to practice circumcision and the operation is depicted in a relief from around 2345 B.C.E. on the doorway to the tomb in the city of Memphis of Ankh-Ma-Hor, vizier of King Teti, the only surgical operation depicted in Egyptian art. This operation was likely performed as a ritual initiation into manhood, or as an initiation ceremony for the *hem-ka* priests, rather than for medical reasons. It is not clear why Ankh-ma-hor might have wanted this scene in his tomb, or if it is supposed to depict his own circumcision. In either case, evidence from mummies indicates that the operation was normally performed in late puberty and it was not done to all male members of the social classes who were mummified. The practice was probably introduced to the Hebrews during their bondage in Egypt, for whom it signified the covenant between the Hebrew people and the Lord (as explained in Genesis 17:10–14). Another scene in the Bible describes Moses's wife, Zipporah, cutting off the foreskin of their son with a sharp flint stone while journeying from Midian to Egypt (Exodus 4:25–26).

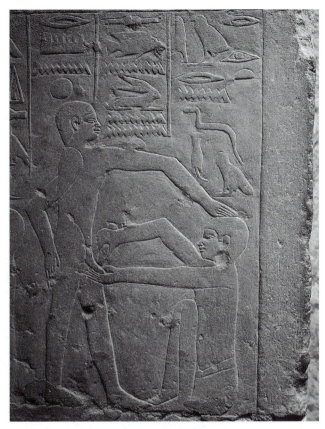

This relief from the Mastaba of Ankh-Ma-Hor, *The Doctor's Tomb*, depicts a youth being circumcised. This is the oldest known depiction of a circumcision, from the Egyptian sixth dynasty in the Old Kingdom (ca. 2350–2200 B.C.E.). (Giraudon/The Bridgeman Art Library)

### Children and Medicine in Ancient Greece and Rome

Greek and Roman medical texts also expressed concern for the differentiated treatment of children and especially the care of newborns. Some, like the Roman Pliny the Elder (23–79 C.E.), provided advice that mixed naturalistic medicinal remedies with amulets and magical cures. For example, Pliny explained, "The tooth of a wolf tied on as an amulet keeps away childish terrors and ailments due to teething, as does also a piece of wolf's skin. . . . The brain of a she-goat, passed through a golden ring, is given drop by drop by the Magic to babies, before they are fed with milk, to guard them from epilepsy and other diseases of babies" (Jones 1963, 173–175). By contrast, the physician Soranus of Ephesus (fl. 100 C.E.) focused more on offering naturalistic medical advice. He wrote a treatise on gynecology in Greek in which he dedicated several chapters to the appropriate treatment of newborns. He describes how to sever the umbilical cord, how to breastfeed and wean the infant, how one should swaddle a baby, and how to teach it to walk so as to promote the proper development and shape of the limbs. Betraying his own biases, Soranus notes that in Rome people were more likely to mishandle these essential childrearing tasks, "for the women in this city do not possess sufficient devotion to look after everything as the purely Grecian women do" (Temkin 1956, 116). Other chapters focus specifically on the treatment of certain infant and childhood medical conditions, including teething, thrush, inflamed tonsils, and illnesses causing coughs and diarrhea. Furthermore, Soranus explains how one should select an appropriate wet nurse, taking into account not only the state of her breasts and supply of milk, but also her character, "since by nature the nursling becomes similar to the nurse and accordingly grows sullen if the nurse is ill-tempered, but of mild disposition if she is even-tempered. . . . For the same reason the wet nurse should not be superstitious and prone to ecstatic states so that she may not expose the infant to danger when led astray by fallacious reasoning, sometimes even trembling like mad" (Temkin 1956, 93).

Soranus also draws attention to the practice of exposure or child abandonment in the ancient Greek and Roman worlds. He writes,

> The majority of barbarians, as the Germans and Scythians, and even some of the Hellenes [i.e., Greeks], put the newborn into cold water in order to make it firm and to let die, as not worth rearing, one that cannot bear the chilling but becomes livid or convulsed. . . . We, however, reject all of these. For cold, on account of its strong and sudden condensing action the like of which the child has not experienced, harms all; and though the harm resulting from the cold escapes notice in those more resistant it is, on the other hand, demonstrated by those susceptible to disease when they are seized by convulsions and apoplexies. Certainly, the fact that the child did not withstand the injury does not prove that it was impossible for it to live if unharmed; more resistant children will also thrive better if not harmed in any way. (Temkin 1956, 82)

Despite his misgivings about this harsh treatment, Soranus begins his account of the care of newborns by explaining how to recognize "whether it is worth rearing or not" based on whether it was deemed strong enough to survive. The Greek author Polybius (ca. 203–120 B.C.E.) had previously noted that some Greek families tried to limit themselves to having only one or two children and Aristotle (384–322 B.C.E.) implied that employing contraceptives or abortifacients to control family size was acceptable so long as they were used prior to the formation of the fetus (which he believed occurred in the middle of the second trimester). Soranus's advice reveals that exposure, abandoning weak or sickly infants in the wilderness, was also a common method for preventing family growth in the ancient world. Plutarch (ca. 46–ca. 120 C.E.), a Greek historian, makes it clear that this custom was regularly practiced by the Spartans, who wished to raise only those who would become strong warriors, but it was likely common throughout the Greek and Roman world.

The ultimate decision in both the Greek and Roman worlds as to whether to raise the child rested with the father. In both cultures, ceremonies were held some days after the birth in which the baby was revealed to the community, symbolically marking its acceptance into the family. In Athens, a ritual called the *amphidromia* was held on the seventh day after birth, which entailed performing sacrifices to the gods followed by a ceremony in which the father carried the infant through the doorway to the house, which would often be decorated with wool for a girl and with an olive garland for a boy, and placed it before the household hearth. Similarly, in Rome on the eighth day after birth for a girl and the ninth day after birth for a boy the ritual of the *dies lustricus* (purification day) was held in which the mother and child were both purified and the child was given a name, marking its acceptance into the family.

## Pediatric Care in the Ayurvedic Tradition

Ayurvedic medical texts contain extensive information devoted to the care of infants and children. According to the *Susruta Samhita* and the *Caraka Samhita*, immediately after birth the newborn should be cleansed and its mouth should be washed with a mixture of rock salt and clarified butter, after which the umbilical cords should be cut. The postnatal ceremony of *jatakarman* would also be performed in which the infant is given an electuary of honey, butter, some plant juices, and powdered gold with the recitation of specific mantras, to provide intelligence, long life, and strength to the baby. In the following days, a series of further rituals would be performed to protect the infant and mother from demons; the room in which they slept would be strewn with various aromatic substances (crushed sesame seed, mustard, and linseed), a purifying fire would be maintained to fumigate the chamber, and a Brahman would perform atonement prayers for ten days, during which time friends and relatives were expected to keep watch, sing songs, and do their best to create a cheerful environment. Furthermore, a bundle of twigs and plants called *raksoghna* (demon-killing) was to be tied above the door to the room and also placed on the child's body to ward off evil spirits. On the tenth day after birth, the woman was allowed to rise from bed, and the naming ceremony (*namakarana*) would take place in which the child would receive its popular name and another name, derived from the constellation at the time of its birth. In the months after birth, further ceremonies were performed: in the fourth month the "first going out" rite (*niskramana*) occurred, when the child was dressed in fine clothes and taken out of the room to worship the gods, then in the sixth to eighth month a physician would make a hole in its earlobes (in the right ear first for boys, the left ear first for girls) from which golden rings would be hung.

The *Caraka* has further advice on how the child's room should be constructed and furnished. The author emphasizes that it should be well ventilated, filled with sunlight, fumigated with aromatic substances and kept clean and free of insects. In addition to attending to the child's physical environment, the *Caraka* also expresses concern for attending to the child's emotional well-being. Appropriate toys are described, with emphasis on making them safe and entertaining: they should be colorful, produce fun noises, be easy to handle, and not be too heavy, sharp, or otherwise dangerous or frightening. Furthermore, the author urges parents to take precautions against frightening the child by wakening it suddenly or handling it violently and not to threaten it with demons even when it is disobedient or become angry when it cries or does not eat, lest this disturb the balance of the *doshas* in the body, making it vulnerable to demonic possession.

Possession by demons was believed to be one of the greatest threats to the health of infants and children. Symptoms of demonic possession included fever, crying, biting the nurse, vomiting, inability to sleep soundly, diarrhea, hoarseness, and loss of appetite. The *Susruta* describes nine different *grahas*, demons that caused disease in children, especially those children who lived in an unclean environment, with dirty wet nurses, or those who are angry, frightened, or in a bad mood. Thus, the precautions described in the *Caraka* for the careful maintenance of the room and toys for children can be seen as a means of warding off the threat of *grahas* and other evil spirits. In addition to managing the child's living space, certain medicines, baths, sacrifices, and invocations are called for to drive out demons from those children who are possessed.

Ayurvedic medical texts also attribute children's diseases to the influence of the mother's or nurse's milk. Thus, the *Susruta* explains,

A child nursed at the breast of any and every woman for want of a nurse of the commendable type, may fall an easy prey to disease owing to the fact of the promiscuous nature of the milk proving uncongenial to its physical temperament. The milk of a nurse not being pressed out and spelled off at the outset may produce cough, difficulty of breathing, or vomiting of the child, owing to the sudden rush of the accumulated milk into its throat choking up the channels. Hence a child should not be allowed to suck in such milk. (Bhishagratna 1911, 227)

The wet nurse was supposed to be chaste, to come from a good family of the same caste as the infant's family, and to have a living male child of her own. The nurse was also expected to attend to her hygiene and diet to ensure that her milk would not become unhealthy. Bad milk could induce the derangement of the *doshas* in the child leading to various diseases, such as *ksiralasaka* (milk-tympany), a disease recognized by watery, frothy and bad-smelling diarrhea, white-yellow and sticky urine, fever, vomiting, and flatulence.

## Pediatrics in Traditional Chinese Medicine

The earliest medical texts in traditional Chinese medicine, like the *Huangdi Neiching*, do not give much attention to the diseases or treatment of children as distinct from general medicine. The development, however, of a meritocratic system of advancement for civil and military officials during the Han dynasty (206 B.C.E.–220 C.E.), which highlighted the need to educate young boys in preparation for future government service, drew increased attention to children and childhood. Han leaders called for the establishment of a public school system and numerous books were written to advise mothers on the best methods of child-rearing and early childhood education. One of these texts even declared "learning begins in the womb" and offered advice on appropriate activities for pregnant women to prepare their fetus while it was still in the uterus. The education of girls received far less attention since they would not have been able to assume public duties in the military or in the civil service.

The *Book of Rites*, compiled originally by Confucius (551–479 B.C.E.) and re-edited during the Han dynasty, describes a number of rules or rituals for conduct, including passages concerning the incorporation of newborn children into the family, and rituals to mark the growing development of the child and its relation to the family. According to the text, the mother and newborn were to be confined to a separate room until the third day after birth when a divinatory ceremony, including necessary sacrifices and rituals, would be held to identify a good man (not the father), who would receive the child and carry him out of the birth chamber to his bedroom. After three months, another ritual was held in which the child's hair would be shaved off (leaving certain portions, depending on whether it was a boy or girl) and then it would be taken from the bedchamber and presented to the father, who would only then give the child a name. These rituals recognize the gradual introduction of the child into the family and public life. Other celebratory rituals, like the hair-pinning and capping of teenage boys and girls and marriage rituals, marked the child's further progress into later life stages (adolescence and adulthood).

These developments regarding views of children during the Han period likely stimulated growing medical interest in the treatment of children. Under the Sui dynasty (581–618 C.E.) and more so under the Tang dynasty (618–907 C.E.), the specialized field of pediatric medicine (*erke*) developed rapidly. The physician Sun Simiao (581–682 C.E.) devoted a chapter in his *Qianjin Yaofang* (*Prescriptions of the Thousand Ounces of Gold*) to maternal and infantile disorders. Declaring that nothing was more important than raising children well, Sun Simiao described appropriate methods for bathing infants, selecting wet nurses, and regulating feeding. Reflecting the growing interest in diseases of children, the Imperial Medical Academy during the Tang dynasty created a new department of pediatrics for training specialized pediatricians. Pediatric medicine took greater steps during the Song dynasty (960–1279 C.E.) and Yuan dynasty (1271–1368 C.E.). The physician Qian Yi (1035–1117 C.E.) devoted forty years of his life to the treatment of children, and his student Yan Xiaozhong recorded his observations in the *Xiao'er Yaozheng Zhijue* (*The Appropriate Way of Recognizing and Treating Infant Maladies*), which focused on the physiological, pathological, and therapeutic aspects of pediatric medicine. Among other things, Qian Yi distinguished between the symptoms and treatment of measles, chickenpox, and smallpox. He viewed smallpox as a disease of children (reflecting the fact that it was an endemic disease in China by this time) and described it in particular as being produced by a fetal toxin, passed from parents to children. He also developed specialized medical formulas for use in treating children, emphasizing that they required different treatment than adults. His book was followed by a number of other texts focused on pediatric medicine, reflecting the fact that this field was well established during the Song dynasty.

The philosopher Han Fei Tzu (ca. 280–233 B.C.E.) observed that it was common in his day for couples to expose infant girls rather than raise them. Laws from the Qin dynasty against infanticide confirm this practice.

In a legal text from 217 B.C.E., we learn that parents had the right to kill newborns that were deformed, but the law did not condone infanticide when "the child's body is whole and without deformity [and the child is killed] merely because [the parents] have too many children and do not wish it to live" (McLeod and Yates 1981, 151). Later texts also denounce infanticide. In the mid-seventh century C.E., the *Nan Shi* (*History of the Southern Dynasties*) reports that the governor of Ren Fang passed a law declaring that parents who refused to bring up their child should be judged as if they had committed murder. These condemnations likely reflect a desire to maintain a strong population to protect imperial power. Nonetheless, other sources suggest that child abandonment and infanticide were prevalent in ancient China. Indeed, the *Yili* (*Book of Etiquette and Ceremonial*), a Confucian compilation on social rituals composed during the Han dynasty, discusses mourning rituals for children, recognizing different procedures depending upon the age of the child when it died. For those that died between the ages of three months and seven years it indicates that the parents should wear no mourning garments; it implies through silence that those who die when younger than three months of age (prior to being received and named by the father) would not be mourned at all. Given these accounts it appears likely that child abandonment and infanticide was common in China, as in other parts of the ancient world.

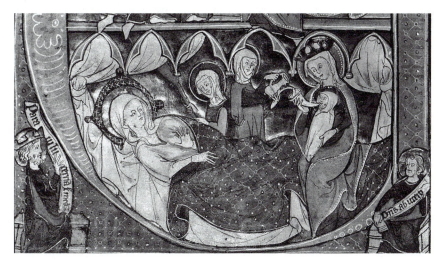

In this thirteenth-century French manuscript illustration a mother is shown in bed attended by another woman. On the right two women use a cow's horn to feed her infant. (Wellcome Library, London)

## Childcare and Pediatric Medicine in Medieval Europe

Medieval Europe witnessed a dramatic increase in the number of texts concerned with childcare and childhood from the twelfth to the fifteenth centuries. Medical texts also gave greater attention to the specific medical needs of children and the treatment of childhood diseases. The proliferation of these writings reflects the importance given to providing for the physical, psychological, and spiritual well-being of children during this period, both among church leaders and the wider community in general. In fact, the vast attention given to children in this period challenges some earlier historical scholarship suggesting that people did not value children or the concept of childhood during the Middle Ages.

Physicians wrote extensively on infant and child health care, not only within their more general medical manuals but also in treatises dedicated specifically to child and infant care, such as the *Practica puerorum in cunabulis* (*Practical Manual on Children in Cradles*) and the *De passionibus puerorum* (*On the Diseases of Children*). The physician Michele Savonarola (1385–1468) recognized that the treatment of infants and children presented a distinct challenge because the patients were often unable to articulate their complaints, making the task of diagnosis more difficult, and, furthermore, he felt that the normal diagnostic measures of taking the pulse and studying the urine were not as useful in children since they were smaller and their bodies behaved differently. Savonarola and other authors recognized a wide range of diseases specific to children such as *marasmus* (what we might recognize as a severe form of malnutrition), which was believed to be caused by the untimely consumption of the body's radical moisture (*humidum radicale*). Other conditions like "*parvitas corporis*" (achondroplasia or dwarfism), smallpox, and measles were also described as children's diseases, along with a wide range of conditions causing vomiting, wheezing, coughing, and fevers. Cures were always supposed to be gentle, and bloodletting and cautery were deemed inappropriate, especially for infants. There were also many remedies to stop infants from crying, like the magical-astrological cure of putting an image of Capricorn on the infant's navel; the best remedy, however, was nursing—hence why Savonarola called the nurse's nipple the "baby-pacifier."

The authors of medical texts did not limit themselves to offering medical advice about disease; they also discussed different aspects of childrearing and some even addressed the appropriate moral education of children. Physicians, following their Greek sources, offered advice on the selection of wet nurses but advocated that mothers should nurse their own children; Bernard de Gordon (active in the late thirteenth and early fourteenth centuries) complained that "women nowadays are too delicate or too haughty, or they do not like the inconvenience" of nursing their own children (Demaitre 1977, 474). They also offered advice on how and when children should be weaned. Savonarola, for example, argued that boys should be weaned at around age three, six months to a year later than girls, because, he said, males live longer than females. Other physicians suggested that in order to encourage weaning the mother or wet nurse should apply unpleasant substances like mustard to their nipples, although many indicated that this could be dangerous and warned that one should not wean a child too suddenly. Finally, medical texts that considered children's health also frequently discussed methods for teaching them how to walk, speak, and learn good manners.

Numerous accounts of divine intervention or miraculous cures for children survive, providing insight into the kinds of dangers they faced. According to these accounts, children received miraculous cures for a wide range of illnesses or disabilities, indicating the extent to which they were susceptible to disease and confirming modern impressions of the high infant mortality for this period. In many cases, children, especially those under the age of six, received miracle cures after having been injured in the course of normal childhood activities rather than for diseases (e.g., drowning, burns, choking or suffocation, fractures, lacerations). Older children faced dangers not only from play, but also from working with adults alongside large farm animals in fields, or in the course of performing other chores, such as collecting firewood or water.

Records of miracle cures may suggest that young boys and girls were often poorly supervised, but they also make clear the extent to which parents loved their children. Parents would go to great lengths to achieve a miracle cure for their children, often taking the child on an extended pilgrimage in order to pray at a saint's shrine. Many saints were known for curing children, but the story of Saint Guinefort is especially surprising. According to legend, a greyhound that had been defending his child from attackers was unjustly killed by its master, who thought the dog had been trying to harm the child. Peasants in the nearby region learned of this event and began to venerate the dog as a saint, Saint Guinefort, and brought their ailing children from miles around to pray at his "shrine," and they reported many successful cures. The cult of Saint Guinefort continued to thrive in the thirteenth century, despite efforts by the church to denounce the veneration of the dog as sacrilegious superstition.

In the thirteenth and fourteenth centuries it became common practice to have infants baptized soon after birth, replacing previous practice of performing baptisms only twice per year. The religious ceremony of baptism performed by a priest marked the formal, public recognition of the child and its entry into the Christian community. The religious belief that anyone who died without being baptized would not be accepted into heaven placed particular importance on performing this ritual soon after birth. Indeed, recognizing the dangers facing unbaptized children, Church authorities even allowed midwives to perform emergency baptisms (even in utero) when it appeared that the child would not survive the birth process. As the child grew, other sacraments marked different life stages, such as confirmation when the child reached adolescence and then the sacrament of marriage marking entry into adulthood.

Although infanticide and child abandonment were practiced in medieval Europe, parents still often expressed a concern for the survival of the child's soul. One story from the fifteenth century recounts the desperate case of a young woman named Denisette Bieart, who gave birth in a courtyard outside an inn and after delivering a daughter, "went into the inn, where she took a basin and water . . . and having done this she climbed up to the privies, and there she took the said child by one of its arms and threw the water on its head, saying, "My child, I baptize you in the name of the Father, the Son, and the Holy Spirit". . . and then threw her child in the privies of the inn" (Park 2010, 25–26). This account of infanticide reminds us of the importance of baptism in medieval society; indeed, a mother could face harsher penalties for killing an unbaptized child. More typical accounts tell of children abandoned on church steps or outside monasteries. In many of these cases, the child was left with a little bag of salt, which served as an indication that the child had not yet been baptized and as payment for its baptism. These stories reflect the general hope that the child would survive and be raised elsewhere, even if the parents could not afford to raise it themselves.

## GERIATRIC CARE IN THE PREMODERN WORLD

If a person managed to survive the dangers associated with childhood, he or she would have a much higher chance of surviving to old age. Indeed, those with adequate nutrition and who did not lead especially dangerous lives might live for a long time—the ancient Egyptian kings Pepi II and Ramses II, for example, lived well into their eighties. Nonetheless, it does appear that few people in premodern societies lived to sixty, let alone eighty years of age. Medical texts from early cultures,

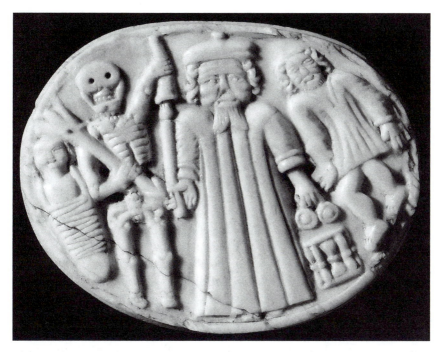

This is an ivory carved spectacle case from around 1500. Spectacles were in use in Europe from the early thirteenth century, and Roger Bacon discussed the scientific principles behind the use of corrective lenses for the elderly in his *Opus Majus* (ca. 1266). The carved case cover shows man in the different stages of life: infancy (the swaddled infant on the left), middle age (the man on the right) and old age (the physician in his academic gown in the middle). The elderly physician is shown holding a pair of spectacles. The hour glass (shown beneath the spectacles) is a reminder of the flow of time leading from infancy to old age. The figure of death, holding a disease arrow, appears to claim the elderly physician, symbolically snuffing out his candle. (Wellcome Library, London)

however, do still consider the effects of aging and offer remedies to hide or slow the onset of old age. The Ebers papyrus in Egypt, for example, describes a number of remedies for turning grey hairs black and for growing hair on a bald head and there are several incantations in Mesopotamian medical texts for the same procedures. The remedies directed at the elderly may not have been as common as remedies for children, but some authors did perceive the need to provide cures for problems brought on by old age.

In India and China, physicians considered a variety of means by which one could delay the onset of old age, especially with the application of alchemical medicine. The Taoist tradition in China, for example, often discussed the alchemical preparation of cinnabar, which produced a series of transformations in its substance, each of which had a magical or medical value.

> At the first transmutation, it is called *Cinnabar Flower*. Heated in a sealed reaction-vessel for thirty-six days, this cinnabar, mixed with mercury, can be turned into gold.
> At the second transmutation, it is called *Divine Talisman*. If one coats the soles of his feet with this cinnabar, he can walk on water or cross through fire. It expels worms from the body and heals all illness. . . .
> At the seventh transmutation, it is called *Weak* [or *Infant*] *Cinnabar*. After one hundred days, one becomes immortal. Even those who are ninety years old can beget children. (Schipper 1993, 177)

The ultimate goal of achieving the status of "immortal," which is equated with the quest for rejuvenation in the Taoist tradition, placed great emphasis on producing elixirs to prolong life or restore the signs of youth. In the Siddha tradition in the tenth century, *rasayana* (medicines designed to increase vigor, improve memory, and otherwise restore youth) were prepared through the process of alchemy and mostly prescribed metallic and mineral substances such as mercury. By contrast, in the Ayurvedic tradition, represented by the *Caraka Samhita*, *rasayana* were usually herbal medicines, but intended for the same effect.

In medieval Europe, some physicians and natural philosophers wrote about remedies for the consequences of aging. Roger Bacon's (ca. 1214–1294) books, *De retardatione accidentium senectutis* (*On the Delay of the Consequences of Old Age*) and *De conservanda iuventute* (*On the Preservation of Youth*), both provided advice for prolonging vitality. Books offering medical advice for old age did not always circulate widely and were often written specifically to offer advice on diet and regimen to a single patron, who was approaching what was viewed as the age of decline. For example, Guido da Vigevano (ca. 1280–ca. 1349) wrote a text specifically for King Philip VI of France in 1335 with a section specifically on "the preservation of health of the old," which was not widely copied or distributed, while the physician Sigismund Albich (1347–1427) wrote a text with advice on the care of old age for King Wenceslas IV of Bohemia. Some texts on geriatric medicine did find a wider circulation, however; Gabriele Zerbi's (1445–1505) *Gerontocomia*, written for Pope Innocent VIII, achieved fame as the first printed text on old age and reached a much wider audience.

The medical authors recognized a series of conditions related to aging, such as Roger Bacon's catalog:

> Grey hair, paleness and wrinkling of the skin, weakness of the faculties and powers, diminution of the blood and spirits, bleariness of the eyes, abundance of mucus, putrid spittle, weakness of breathing, insomnia, anger and mental restlessness, and lesion of the instruments of the senses in which [the faculties of the brain work]. (Demaitre 1990, 10)

To treat these concerns, physicians typically focused on regulating the individual's diet and regimen in order to sustain the physical and mental faculties. Medicinal elixirs and occult remedies that could "prolong life" also formed part of the physician's repertoire for managing old age. Many of these prescriptions were expected to work by sympathetic magic; for example, one cure called for eating agaric, a white fungus, to purge the phlegm of the elderly because it had the same color as phlegm. Some elixirs for prolonging life reflect the influence of alchemical thought. Tommaso Rangoni of Ravenna (1493–1577) summarized the ingredients of many such elixirs described in previous texts, describing their occult or hidden properties, when writing for three successive popes on how to prolong their lives. He said that the three most successful occult ingredients were gold, pearls, and "square stone of the noble animals" (*lapis quadratus nobilis animalis*) since they had the power to retard the loss of the radical moisture (*humidum radicale*). Other popular ingredients in the elixirs for prolonging life were rosemary, aloewood, viper's flesh (the main ingredient in theriac), "bone of stag's heart," and *aqua vite* (distilled wine). Finally, we should note one of the most significant contributions for the elderly from the Middle Ages: Roger Bacon, who was interested in the science of optics, is also credited with inventing eyeglasses to help those with declining vision.

# CHAPTER 6

# Infectious Disease in the Premodern World

## STUDYING DISEASE IN HISTORY

Studying the patterns of infectious diseases in the premodern world is fraught with difficulties. Paleopathologists offer some insight into the prevalence of diseases in early societies by observing signs of pathological lesions in human skeletal remains, yet only chronic, degenerative diseases (e.g., tuberculosis, leprosy, and syphilis) leave visible evidence of infection in hard tissues that can be studied today; individuals who die from an infectious disease typically do so long before the condition could cause deformation in teeth or bones. These efforts are further complicated by the fact that it is not always easy to know with certainty which disease may have caused a particular pathological lesion. Recent advances in techniques to extract DNA samples from human remains (e.g., from surviving dental pulp tissue or mummified remains) have made it possible to look for signs of other infectious organisms that do not otherwise cause damage to hard tissues (e.g., finding the DNA for the agents causing diseases such as bubonic and pneumonic plague or smallpox). Nonetheless, these techniques still only allow a fragmentary picture of the patterns of disease in early societies.

Another means of learning about the incidence of infectious diseases in premodern societies is to examine the written evidence. Interpreting premodern accounts of disease presents its own challenges, however. These accounts do not always list enough specific symptoms to allow modern physicians to make a clear diagnosis of what the disease may have been. A case in point is the disease *di'u*, described in ancient Mesopotamia as being a summer affliction characterized by fevers, sweating, and headaches. Based on the general symptoms, we might associate *di'u* with a range of different infectious diseases, parasitic diseases such as malaria, or with heat stroke. Thus, Mesopotamians seem to have recognized a range of conditions under the heading of a single disease entity, *di'u*, whereas modern physicians would wish to distinguish among them. When looking at diseases in history, differential diagnosis, the systematic practice of discerning the specific cause of a disease from a number of related possibilities, is further complicated by difficulties in translation or understanding what is meant by specific words, like the reference to "Khonsu's tumor" (*aat net Khonsu*) discussed in the Egyptian Ebers papyrus; different scholars have translated this phrase variously to describe bubonic plague buboes, the growths associated with tubercular leprosy, or possibly cancer. Thus, accurately determining disease patterns in the premodern world based on the written evidence is not always possible.

For historians of medicine, the task of identifying the actual disease described in the written records is often less important than trying to learn how a disease was understood in a given society and how that might shape an individual's experience of illness. With these goals in mind, it is worth considering the comparative theories of disease in different cultures and the social responses to some specific diseases within those cultures. Epidemic diseases posed a constant threat, and a variety of plagues spread regularly through premodern societies. Smallpox and bubonic plague rank among the most deadly epidemic diseases in world history, and they elicited a variety of responses in different cultures. Although it did not claim as many lives as smallpox or bubonic plague, leprosy was prevalent throughout premodern societies and created its own set of challenges. In this chapter we will consider the medical and social responses to these diseases in world history.

## EPIDEMICS AND THEORIES
## OF DISEASE CAUSATION

Premodern societies had a number of ways for explaining the cause and process of disease in a single person. A range of explanations might be offered to account for the onset of disease in an individual, including the role of personal sin, invading demons or evil spirits, or

inadequate diet and regimen. These theories, however, could not easily explain why hundreds and thousands of people could all suddenly
fall ill and die at around the same time, while exhibiting the same
symptoms. The sudden appearance and rapid spread of epidemic disease within a large population requires a different explanation for how
disease spreads that not only accounts for the nature of an individual
body but also makes clear why multiple people would be infected by
the same ailment.

Today we are accustomed to thinking of the multiple vectors by which
diseases can be transmitted. In the face of fears of a possible deadly
influenza pandemic, the spread of viruses like HIV and SARS (severe
acute respiratory syndrome), and the rise of drug-resistant strains of
bacteria causing infectious diseases like tuberculosis, we are continually reminded of the dangers of contagion, the human-to-human transmission of disease. Despite the fact that people in premodern societies
no doubt recognized that certain diseases could be transmitted from a
sick person to a healthy one, in general theories of contagion played
only a minor role in early explanations for the spread of disease. Even
in cases in which premodern people employed terminology to express
a concept of contagion, they did not necessarily conceive of the mechanisms of transmission in the way that we do today, that is, by touch or
other contact with an infected person that could pass along a "germ."
In the Greek world, Galen of Pergamum (129–ca. 216 C.E.) was well
aware of the fact that some diseases could be caught from other sufferers and considered the possibility of "seeds" of disease that could
be transmitted between people, but he did not give much weight to
it in his considerations on the spread of disease and the concept was
not developed in later Roman, Islamic, or medieval European medical
writings that built upon the Greek philosophical tradition. Likewise,
Chinese and Indian medical texts reflect an awareness of diseases that
can be transmitted by human-to-human contact, but place far greater
emphasis on other explanations for the spread of disease.

Healers in premodern societies generally did not believe that contagion was sufficient to explain how so many people could acquire
the same illness so swiftly. Most often, doctors emphasized the role
of environmental factors when discussing the cause and rapid spread
of epidemic disease. The Greek Hippocratic text, *Airs, Waters, Places,*
examined the different diseases that might be caused by seasonal
changes, different winds (depending on the direction of the winds and
whether they are hot or cold), proximity to bodies of water (e.g., spring
waters vs. marshlands and swamps), or by other astronomical and
meteorological factors. The author claims that attending to these factors

will allow the physician "to tell what epidemic diseases will attack the city either in summer or in winter. . . . For knowing the changes of the seasons, and the risings and settings of the stars, with the circumstances of each of these phenomena, he will know beforehand the nature of the year that is coming" (Jones 1984, 73). Building upon these ideas, Greek physicians developed the theory of miasmas, fetid or corrupted airs, which could arise in a region and cause many people to contract the same disease in a short period of time by adversely affecting everybody's humoral balance. Traditional Chinese medicine and Ayurvedic medicine also attributed the spread of epidemic diseases to the negative effects environmental factors might have on people's bodily systems. The *Huangdi Neiching* (*The Yellow Emperor's Classic of Internal Medicine*), for example, offered the following advice:

> Huang Di asked, "As extremes and disharmonies occur during the interplay of the natural elements, plagues and disease arise to cause suffering in people. What are the ways that can help to prevent the effects of imbalance from the macrocosm upon human beings?"
>
> Qi Bo replied, "You have asked a question that deserves an answer in depth. Generally, a physician needs to be versed in the laws of the universe and its interactive dynamics, and to have a firm grasp of the knowledge of acupuncture, in order to know when to fortify a deficient and when to reduce an excessive state and how to maintain constancy of energy flow in patients." (Ni 1995, 273)

Therefore, doctors needed to known how to counteract the adverse effects of the environmental factors by fortifying the body through changes in diet and regimen, or through other means such as the use of prophylactic acupuncture or bloodletting.

Epidemic diseases were also regularly attributed to divine or supernatural causes in premodern sources. In the Ayurvedic tradition, the *Susruta Samhita* categorizes diseases according to their various causes and details a range of causes for epidemic diseases:

> Sometimes a town or a city is depopulated by a curse, anger, sin, or by a monster or a demoness conjured up by a spell or incantation. Sometimes the pollens of poisonous flowers or grasses, etc., wafted by the winds, invade a town or a village, and produce a sort of epidemic cough, asthma, catarrh, or fever, irrespective of all constitutional peculiarities or deranged bodily humors agitated thereby. Towns and villages are known to have been depopulated through malignant astral influences, or through houses, wives, beds, seats, carriages, riding animals, gems and precious stones assuming inauspicious features. (Bhishagratna 1907, 52)

This full range of both environmental and supernatural explanations for epidemic disease is followed by a similarly wide range of therapeutic advice, including the use of drugs, but with special emphasis on performing rituals of purification and penance, praying and making sacrificial offerings to the gods, showing self-control, kindness and obedience to elders, and following other such rules of conduct which "may prove beneficial to the affected community" (Bhishagratna 1907, 52). Clearly, epidemic diseases could be explained in many ways and responses to them varied.

## SMALLPOX

The earliest evidence for the origins of smallpox come from ancient Egypt and the Indus Valley; significantly, three mummies from the Eighteenth and Twentieth dynasties in Egypt (1570–1085 B.C.E.), including the pharaoh Ramses V (d. 1157 B.C.E.), show marked signs of pustular eruptions indicative of smallpox. Smallpox, caused by the *variola major* virus, had a mortality rate of 25 to 30 percent, and it was, therefore, especially feared. Those who survived acquired a natural immunity to the disease and so would not be subject to repeat infection. Consequently, the natural history of smallpox suggests that it probably did not exist until the rise of civilizations with sufficient populations to sustain it. After an initial incubation period of roughly twelve days, people infected by the disease would develop a high fever, headaches, and body pains, followed by the eruption of a distinctive rash developing first on the face before spreading over the arms, chest, back, and legs. The rash itself would give rise to raised pimples, then blisters, and then pustules, which dried up and turned into scabs. Those who died from the disease typically did so within three to five days, but others could succumb to complications attributed to the disease eighteen days or more after the first symptoms appeared. Survivors were often left with pockmarked faces and sometimes were blinded in one or both eyes. The high mortality coupled with the danger of permanent disfiguration for survivors made this a particularly fearsome disease in the premodern world.

Hindu mythology suggests that smallpox was likely present in India at roughly the same time as in Egypt. Religious texts make numerous allusions to the worship of Shitala, the goddess of smallpox, who was supposed to possess the body of individuals, thereby causing the disease. The *Atharvaveda* also describes a series of services and prayers that Brahmin priests would offer for the worship of Shitala, which included a ritual of inoculation in which people would breathe in dried scabs from smallpox lesions to induce a mild case of the disease. These unsystematic rituals likely led to the death of many and were probably not effective enough to have thwarted large-scale outbreaks of the disease, but they offer the earliest account of inoculation measures in the world. The practice of inoculating against smallpox was later introduced into China from India during the Sung dynasty (960–1279 C.E.), where the procedure was known as "planting the flowers" since the Chinese often called smallpox pustules the "Heavenly Flowers." The earliest medical description of *masurika*, or smallpox, in the Ayurvedic tradition is found in the *Susruta Samhita*, which describes the disease as being caused by a derangement of the *doshas*. Later medical texts continued to develop diagnostic accounts of the disease, offering a range of diet, drugs, and other forms of therapy designed to correct the imbalances of the *doshas*. Both the naturalistic and divine explanations of the disease coexisted in the Indian tradition and both methods of treatment were followed.

Smallpox likely first entered China in the north with the invading the Huns around 250 B.C.E., shortly before the Chinese had completed the protective barrier of the Great Wall. The second major outbreak entered from the south in 48 or 49 C.E. when the emperor's army went to suppress an uprising in the modern-day Hunan Province where an epidemic was in progress. More than half of the Chinese army died from the disease and the survivors brought the disease back with their prisoners. These epidemics were variously called the "Hun pox," "captive's pox," or "barbarian pox," reflecting the belief that they represented diseases brought to China from the outside world. The Taoist adept Ge Hong (ca. 281–341 C.E.) provides the earliest detailed clinical description of the disease in his *Zhouhou Beijifang* (*Emergency Prescriptions*), noting that, "this [disease] is due to poisonous air. The people say that it was introduced in the reign of Chien Wu when that king was fighting with the Huns at Nang Yang. The name of 'Hun pox' has been given to it" (Hopkins 1983, 104). In 610, Chao Yuanfang compiled a medical text, the *Zhu bing yuan hou fun* (*Compilation on the Origins of Disorders*), in which he explained that the disease was caused by an excessive accumulation of heat toxin in the body, caused by cold damage during the winter or by unseasonal noxious *qi*.

By the Song and Yuan periods (907–1368 C.E.), smallpox was increasingly recognized as a pediatric disorder in China, indicating that it had become endemic so that most adults had already survived exposure to it and were thus immune. Chinese physicians began to attribute the disease to the *tai du* (fetal toxin), a heat toxin introduced into the fetus by way of the mother, father, or both parents—in other words, a hereditary disease. A number of factors were proposed to account for this; for example, the mother's diet, the father's drinking, or the parents continued sexual activity during pregnancy all might elevate the amount of heat toxin in their bodies that could then be passed to the fetus. The *tai du* would remain dormant in the child's body until activated by disorderly climactic conditions, at which point it would spread through the channels of the body and cause smallpox. Recognizing that the disease used not to exist in China, physicians explained that the ancient Chinese forebears had led a purer lifestyle, which had prevented the elevation of heat toxins in their bodies so that they did not contract the disease. By implication, the decadent present-day lifestyle was responsible for the continued spread of smallpox in China and the cure required greater discipline and morality in terms of diet and other behaviors.

Smallpox entered Japan in the sixth century c.e., probably brought by Buddhist missionaries from Korea, who came with statues of the Buddha and several sacred Buddhist books sent as gifts from Korean rulers. Favoring the new religion, Japanese rulers encouraged their subjects to worship the Buddha over their indigenous Shinto gods. The fact that the missions from Korea roughly coincided with the outbreak of smallpox epidemics in Japan led many people to believe that the disease was a punishment for turning away from the Shinto gods. In response, they destroyed the Buddhist statues, burned Buddhist temples, and flogged Buddhist monks and nuns. When the epidemics did not abate, however, others feared that the pestilence was sent as punishment for destroying the images of the Buddha, so later emperors, who converted to Buddhism, erected monasteries and statues of the Buddha to help ward off the disease. In 981 c.e., a Japanese medical book, the *I Shinho*, discussed treatments for those suffering from the disease, advocating isolation in hospitals and wrapping patients in red cloths, or hanging red cloths from the walls of the sickroom as a means of curing the affliction by magical influence.

Although there were likely outbreaks of smallpox in Europe, introduced from Egypt, during the early Greek and Roman periods, the earliest substantive evidence of a smallpox epidemic occurred during the reign of the Roman emperor Marcus Aurelius Antonius in the early third century c.e. Smallpox epidemics are reported in later centuries in Europe, but the population was likely not great enough to support regularly recurring epidemics of the disease until the thirteenth century. Prior to this, the Arabic physician Abu Bakr Muhammad ibn Zakariya al-Razi (d. ca. 925, known as Rhazes in the Latin West) wrote a medical treatise, *On Smallpox and Measles*, in which he distinguished between smallpox and measles for the first time in the Greek medical tradition. By the thirteenth century, several European physicians also described the causes and cures of smallpox in their medical texts, some of whom, like Gilbertus Anglicus in his *Compendium Medicinae* (ca. 1240), advocated treating patients by wrapping them in red blankets in a fashion similar to the practice in Japan. By the fifteenth century, smallpox was increasingly known for afflicting children, suggesting that it had become endemic in Europe by this time, just before European conquerors were to introduce the disease into the Americas.

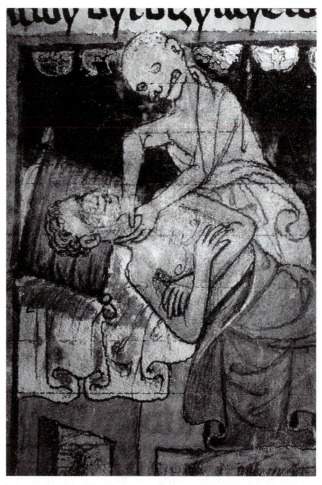

In this European manuscript image from 1376, Death, depicted as a rotting corpse, strangles his next victim. In the years following the first wave of the Black Death, the figure Death was often portrayed in art spreading the plague by shooting plague arrows or dragging away those who died from the disease. (Werner Forman Archive/StockphotoPro)

# BUBONIC PLAGUE, OR THE BLACK DEATH

## The Origin and Spread of the Bubonic Plague

In the mid-fourteenth century C.E. a pandemic spread throughout the Near East, Europe, and North Africa. The disease, known as the Black Death in Europe, is generally assumed to have been bubonic plague caused by the *Yersinia pestis* bacterium. The symptoms could be horrifying, as described by Gabriele de' Mussis (d. 1356) in his *Historia de Morbo*:

> Those of both sexes who were in health, and in no fear of death, were struck by four savage blows to the flesh. First, out of the blue, a kind of chilly stiffness troubled their bodies. They felt a tingling sensation, as if they were being pricked by the points of arrows. The next stage was a fearsome attack which took the form of an extremely hard, solid boil [i.e., plague bubo]. In some people this developed under the armpit and in others in the groin between the scrotum and the body. As it grew more solid, its burning heat caused the patients to fall into an acute and putrid fever, with severe headaches. As it intensified its extreme bitterness could have various effects. In some cases it gave rise to an intolerable stench. In others it brought vomiting of blood, or swellings near the place from which the corrupt humor arose: on the back, across the chest, near the thigh. Some people lay as if in a drunken stupor and could not be roused. Behold the swellings, the warning signs sent by the Lord. All these people were in danger of dying. Some died on the very day the illness took possession of them, others on the next day, others—the majority—between the third and fifth day. There was no known remedy for the vomiting of blood. Those who fell into a coma, or suffered a swelling or the stink of corruption very rarely escaped. But from the fever it was sometimes possible to make a recovery. (Horrox 1994, 24)

The Justinian plague that struck Europe in the mid-sixth century C.E. and described by the Byzantine author Procopius in his *History of the Wars* was likely an outbreak of bubonic plague. Thereafter large bubonic plague epidemics were rare in the West until the Black Death in the fourteenth century, after which the plague was endemic in Europe with near yearly occurrences until the late seventeenth century. Unfortunately, it is difficult to distinguish outbreaks of bubonic plague from other epidemic diseases in Chinese sources, but it seems that the earliest description of bubonic plague in China was by Cha'o Yuan-fang in 610 C.E. and that the disease was endemic in the region between China and India from at least that point forward.

The fourteenth-century pandemic likely originated sometime during the 1330s in the Eurasian steppe, where it had been harbored in populations of burrowing rodents, from where it was carried by Mongol horsemen to other parts of the world. Chinese records suggest that an epidemic swept through the province of Hopei in 1331, killing nine-tenths of the population, and then another epidemic swept more widely through eight different parts of China in 1353–1354 killing up to two-thirds of the population. It seems likely that these epidemics can be tied to the early spread of bubonic plague out of the Eurasian steppe. Otherwise, records reveal little about the spread of the disease in China or into the Indian subcontinent. However, it appeared in the eastern parts of the Muslim world in the mid-1340s, arriving in the Mediterranean by 1347, in Italy, Spain, and southern France by 1348, and in Germany and England by 1349. Estimates suggest that one-quarter to one-third of the population died during this initial wave of the Black Death and thereafter recurrences continued in more localized regions roughly every ten years killing around 10 to 20 percent of the inhabitants with each outbreak.

### Medical Responses to the Black Death in Europe and the Islamic World

Physicians in the Islamic world and in Europe both sought to explain the rapid spread of the plague as a humoral disturbance induced by miasmas, or bad airs; for example, according to one Arabic physician,

> The pestilence resulted from a corruption occurring in the substance of the air due to heavenly and terrestrial causes. In the earth the causes are brackish water and the many cadavers found in places of battle when the dead are not buried, and land which is water-logged and stagnant from rottenness, vermin, and frogs. As regards the heavenly air, the causes are the many shooting stars and meteorites at the end of the summer and in the autumn, the strong south and east winds in December and January, and the signs of rain increase in the winter but it does not rain. (Dols 1977, 88–89)

In Europe, the faculty of medicine at the medical school in Paris explained that an unusual planetary alignment had caused the corruption of airs on earth and induced earthquakes that had released foul vapors from underground. In this way, they tried to account for the sudden onset of this particularly deadly disease in terms of their rational, scientific theories that explained the relationship between the microcosm and the macrocosm. Other physicians also employed the astrological theories to account for the seemingly random way in which the disease spread, affecting some towns and not others, and even seeming to affect people living in one street more than others. One medical astrologer suggested that "each city, town and home has fixed stars and planets ruling it . . . therefore wherever the rules of these places agree in power and effect with the planets and stars bringing the general mortality, those subject to them will have been made ready to receive that celestial influence upon their bodies" (Horrox 1994, 170).

Although, as we have seen, contagion played a minor role in explaining the spread of epidemic disease in the Greek tradition, physicians could not help but recognize that this disease seemed to spread through contact with infected persons. Muslim religious scholars wrote many plague tracts following the initial outbreak of the epidemic, considering the possibility of contagion. Referring to the Prophetic tradition, some scholars maintained that Muhammad had proclaimed that there was no possibility of contagion since this would imply that disease might spread independent of the will of God. However, this issue was complex, and numerous Muslim authors supported the possibility of contagion revealing that there was no single Islamic position on this issue. Ibn al-Khatib (fourteenth century), for example, specifically argued that experience revealed that plague was spread by contagion, and outbreaks often coincided with the arrival of people traveling from regions where the plague was raging. He supported his empirical observations by citing hadith (prophetic sayings) that he felt endorsed the possibility of contagion. The debate over the possibility of contagion continued far beyond the period of the Black Death, but those physicians who supported a contagion theory found it necessary to reconcile it with the miasmatic theory, by arguing, for example, that the sick contaminated the air around them, as well as their clothing, bedding, and utensils. European physicians also sought to reconcile contagion theory with the belief in miasmas. One physician at Montpellier offered a miasmatic explanation of contagion through eye contact with a sick individual:

> But sometimes the brain expels the windy and poisonous matter via the optic nerves at the eyes. This is agony, and the sick man stares fixedly ahead, as if he cannot move his eyes. Amazingly, as it stands in the eyes, the primary windiness assumes the characteristics of a poisonous vapor, and seeks a new home in some other body, which it can enter and be at rest. And if a healthy person sees this visible vapor, he is stamped with the pestilential illness. The man is poisoned faster than air can leave the sick man, for the thin poison moves faster than the heavy air. (Horrox 1994, 183)

The medical response, therefore, focused on mitigating the harmful influences of the miasmas. Most physicians advocated that patients preserve health by regulating their diet and physical activity in order to fortify their bodies against the detrimental affects of the noxious vapors. Another prophylactic measure endorsed by physicians was the use of aromatic substances in a nose pomander or to fumigate rooms in order to cleanse the air. Indeed, the emphasis on miasmas led to efforts to clear cities of the sources of foul smelling air, such as the waste produced by overflowing latrines and butcher shops. Those who fell ill received more direct treatment through bloodletting, cupping, and the administration of drugs, including the much-praised compound medicine, theriac.

### Religious Responses to the Black Death

The dramatic appearance, terrifying symptoms, and high mortality of the plague no doubt gave additional support to arguments for the divine cause of the Black Death. Many Christians viewed the plague in apocalyptic terms, as signifying the end of the world and the coming of Judgment Day when the faithful would be taken into heaven. Similarly, some Islamic theologians described the plague as a mercy and martyrdom for faithful Muslims and a punishment for infidels, relating it to the ideology of the *jihad,* or holy war. However, far greater emphasis was given to the belief that the plague was sent as a divine punishment for individual and communal sin. Several possibilities were offered to explain divine displeasure. In Europe, for example, priests preached from the pulpit about humanity's general sinfulness, but they also identified some specific examples of activities that would merit God's wrath, such as people wearing indecent clothing, women dressing in men's clothes, and disobedient children. Some people responded by pointing to the sins of the clergy as the real reason for divine displeasure.

Belief in the divine origin of the plague led to a number of efforts to restore moral behavior and atone for sin. Religious leaders in many cities in Europe led intercessory processions through the streets or sang special Masses as a means of expressing communal pleas for mercy and atonement for sin. Individuals offered their own prayers, often directed toward the saints specifically recognized for healing those afflicted with plague, Saint Sebastian and Saint Roche. Saint Sebastian was an early Christian who was martyred by Roman soldiers for his faith. According to legend, the soldiers first attempted to execute Sebastian by shooting him with arrows, but he survived this attack and they needed to resort to different means to complete the execution. The arrows themselves were viewed as symbolic of the spread of plague, and by extension Sebastian was known for having survived the assault of the plague, hence why he was considered an appropriate plague saint. Saint Roche, who lived in the fourteenth century, was known for surviving his own infection with the Black Death after which he dedicated his life to caring for other plague victims. Saint Roche is often depicted in artwork raising his robes to reveal the plague bubo in his groin, with the dog that was said to have brought him food while he endured the disease alone in the wilderness.

Another manifestation of religious responses to the plague in Europe was the appearance of groups of laymen and women known as the flagellants, who traveled in processions from town to town, denouncing sinners. During the processions the flagellants would publicly scourge themselves with whips (*flagella*) to atone for the sins of humanity and beg for God's mercy. One witness attests to the ghastly scenes enacted by a troop of flagellants:

> Each whip consisted of a stick with three knotted thongs hanging from the end. Two pieces of needle-sharp metal were run through the center of the knots from both sides, forming a cross, the ends of which extended beyond the knots for the length of a grain of wheat or less. Using these whips they beat and whipped their bare skin until their bodies were bruised and swollen and blood rained down, spattering the walls nearby. I have seen, when they whipped themselves, how sometimes those bits of metal penetrated the flesh so deeply that it took more than two attempts to pull them out. (Horrox 1994, 150)

Although some people were impressed by the flagellants' fervent displays of piety, many members of the clergy were concerned that these actions only revealed the pride and excess of the participants and saw them as a threat to the authority of the church. Ultimately, Pope Clement VI forbade the practice in 1349 and authorities sought, often unsuccessfully, to suppress the flagellant movement in Europe.

### Popular and Civic Responses to the Black Death

In his *Decameron* Giovanni Boccaccio (1313–1375) describes a common response to the appearance of the plague in a city—flight. Citizens refused to help their neighbors and sometimes even deserted members of their own families and, as Boccaccio notes with horror, "even worse, and almost incredible, was the fact that fathers and mothers refused to nurse and assist their own children, as though they did not belong to them" (McWilliam 1995, 8–9). His description vividly portrays the fear evoked by the appearance of the plague.

Driven by fear local inhabitants sometimes identified scapegoats, including foreigners, the poor, and Jews, whom they could blame for the disease. One general accusation was that people were poisoning local wells, thus causing the plague. In cities throughout Europe, many Jews were tortured into confessing to well-poisoning and were burned or otherwise executed for the crime. In response to the merciless massacre of Jews, Pope Clement VI issued a papal bull in 1348 condemning Christians who had falsely accused and impiously slain Jews for spreading the plague and extending papal protection over Jewish communities in Christendom.

Civic and lay authorities also tried to limit the spread of plague. In many towns, lay leaders enacted legislation aimed at cleaning up the source of foul airs in cities, reflecting the prevalence of the belief in miasmatic theory. For example, some cities passed ordinances that banned butchers from dumping the entrails and blood left over from their trade into the streets, since this waste was viewed as a source of corrupt air, and in other cases, tanner's shops were relocated outside city walls—tanners used large, foul-smelling vats of urine in the tanning process. New regulations were also passed requiring that "the bodies of the dead shall not be removed from the place of death until they have been enclosed in a wooden box, and the lid of planks nailed down so that no stench can escape," and that "to avoid the foul stench which comes from dead bodies each grave shall be dug two and a half armslengths deep" (McWilliam 1995, 196). Acknowledging the possibility that the plague was contagious, many cities attempted to establish quarantines, preventing foreigners and linen products from infected regions from entering.

## LEPROSY

Leprosy, or Hansen's disease, is a bacterial infection, which results in skin and nerve damage that can lead to severe disfigurement to the face and deformity of the extremities. The pathogen responsible for Hansen's disease, *Mycobacterium leprae*, may have evolved in East Africa or India before spreading eastward to China and, at a slightly later date, northwest into Europe. Although ancient Mesopotamian and Egyptian medical texts do not provide enough descriptive detail of disease symptoms to positively prove the incidence of leprosy, paleopathologists have discovered skeletons in Egypt that exhibit characteristic symptoms of the disease dating to the second century B.C.E. Indeed, it is often difficult to rely upon premodern diagnoses of "leprosy" since in many cases they are just as likely describing otherwise harmless skin disease like *psoriasis*, as actual cases of Hansen's disease. Greek and Roman authors use a number of terms to identify conditions that might have been leprosy, including the words "lepra" (which means in Greek "a scaly disease") and "elephantiasis" (referring to a disease causing the thickening of the skin and changes to the bones). Likewise, the biblical word "sara'at," which appears thirty-five times in various forms in the Hebrew Old Testament, generally refers to certain skin conditions inflicted on humans for sin (although the term is also applied to house walls and clothing) and has regularly been translated as "leprosy" in the English Bible, although the descriptions do not necessarily support this diagnosis.

## Leprosy in India

In 2009 a team of paleopathologists reported finding evidence of leprosy in the skeletal remains of a middle-aged adult male who lived in India around 2000 b.c.e.—the oldest documented skeletal evidence for leprosy in the world (Robbins et al. 2009). Given that it is not common to find adult burials in this region after 2000 b.c.e., the paleopathologists suggest the burial may imply that it was not considered appropriate to cremate the diseased body as a sacrifice to the Hindu gods. The earliest documentary evidence for this disease in India would seem to confirm this possibility. The condition *kustha*, a dangerous skin condition that has often been thought to be leprosy, is first described in the *Atharvaveda*:

> Born by night art though, O plant, dark, black, sable. Do thou, that art rich in color, stain this leprosy [*kustha*], and the grey spots! . . . The leprosy which has originated in the bones, and that which has originated in the body and upon the skin, the white mark begotten of corruption, I have destroyed with my charm. (Bloomfield 2004, 19)

References to the condition *kustha* are also found in later Hindu religious scriptures, which declare that the disease is a punishment for sinners in their future birth.

Ayurvedic medical texts confirm the religious beliefs about *kustha* found in the *Atharvaveda*, but they also offer a naturalistic explanation that it is caused by a derangement of the *doshas*. The *Susruta Samhita* also suggests that *kustha* is contagious (although the risk of contagion of actual Hansen's disease is slight), transmitted by touch, breath, sexual intercourse, or by sharing utensils, or that it is a hereditary disease passed from parents to offspring. Perhaps unsurprisingly, the remedy reflects a blend of natural and religious measures:

> Wise men hold that, for killing a Brahman, or a woman, or one of his own relations, for theft, as well as for doing acts of impiety, a man is sometimes cursed with this foul disease by way of divine retribution. The disease re-attacks a man even in his next rebirth in the event of his dying with it. Uncured *Kushtham* (leprosy) is the most painful, and most troublesome of all diseases.
>
> A Kushthi (leper), getting rid of this foul malady by observing the proper regimen of diet and conduct and by practicing expiatory penances and by resorting to proper medicinal measures, gets an elevated status after death. (Bhishagratna 1911, 42)

## Leprosy in China

Leprosy was known in China from at least the sixth century B.C.E. in the Zhou dynasty. A bamboo strip containing a number of legal records discovered in a tomb from the third century B.C.E. describes a court case where a doctor was called to confirm whether a person had *li* (leprosy), responding with this diagnosis: "[The villager] has no eyebrows; the bridge of the nose is destroyed; his nasal cavity is collapsed; if you prick his nose, he does not sneeze; . . . the soles of both feet are defective and are suppurating in one place; his hands have no hair; I ordered him to shout and the *ch'i* of his voice was hoarse. It is *li* [leprosy]" (McLeod and Yates 1981, 153). Chinese criminal law from this period indicates that criminals afflicted with *li* could expect a more severe punishment than others convicted of similar offences, including being drowned or buried alive. The different penalties suggest a deeper religious significance attached to those suffering from *li*. Indeed, in this period *li* was associated with possession by a ghastly spirit that personified moral vileness and manifested the external symptoms of the disease on the patient. Thus, burying alive or drowning a criminal afflicted with *li* was a ritual performance to suppress the ghastly spirit. *Li* patients convicted of lesser, non-capital crimes, would still be transferred to special prisons for lepers. Furthermore, those with *li* were deprived of their right to marriage and were often expelled from their communities.

From the fourth through thirteenth centuries C.E., numerous accounts of people suffering from *li* reflect the religious responses to the disease in the Buddhist and Taoist traditions. Stories from the Buddhist tradition emphasize that the disease was a punishment for moral transgressions committed in this life, a former life, or by one's forebears. Buddhist monasteries established special quarters to house *li* sufferers in the sixth and seventh centuries C.E., and many Buddhist monks dedicated their lives to caring from them. For example, around 581 the monk Daoxun was said to travel among those with *li*, selflessly caring for their needs: "Whenever he saw pus flowing out of corrupted sores, he did not have any second thought and cleaned them with his mouth. He washed their clothes, and purified the sins of their hearts" (Leung 2008, 70). In addition to their physical care, Buddhist healers also provided the necessary purification rituals to cleanse the afflicted of their sins. The Taoist tradition, by contrast, places greater emphasis on the role of the sick individual in self-healing by means of practicing bodily and spiritual discipline. The Taoist physician Sun Simiao

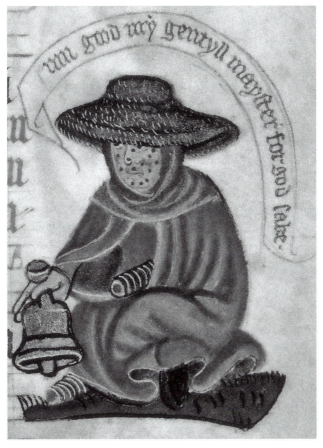

This fourteenth-century European illustration depicts a leper with facial disfigurement and amputated limbs. The leper carries a bell to warn others of her approach. (The British Library/StockphotoPro)

(581–682) spoke of the healing process for *li* in these terms: "There is an auspicious and an inauspicious meaning to this illness. If the sufferer of the disease cultivates good, he will have an auspicious end. If he maintains the same habits as other worldly beings, he will certainly have an inauspicious end" (Leung 2008, 74). Similarly, Taoist stories tell of *li* sufferers who achieved cures by traveling into the mountains and learning to follow a simple spiritual life.

### Leprosy in Medieval Europe

Leprosy entered Western Europe sometime around the fourth century C.E. and spread along expanding mercantile routes and in the developing urban centers. In the twelfth and thirteenth centuries, social and medical responses to leprosy suggest a massive increase in awareness or incidences of the disease. The late fourteenth and fifteenth centuries, by contrast, witness a steep decline in social and medical reports of the disease. This brief upsurge in reports of leprosy in Europe, peaking in the thirteenth century, is difficult to explain. Some scholars have argued that the seeming explosion of leprosy cases represents increased social fear of the disease rather than a real rise in the disease's prevalence. Other explanations suggest that more accurate methods of diagnosis led to fewer people being diagnosed with leprosy in later centuries, or that a greater number of people afflicted by the disease had died as a result of the Black Death due to their weakened immunity, reducing the number of infected individuals. In any event, by the sixteenth century the writings of physicians in Western Europe reflected less concern with leprosy and turned increasingly toward consideration of other diseases such as syphilis.

During the height of leprosy's prevalence in Europe, however, the afflicted often suffered severe social stigmas, as happened in other cultures. Fear that the disease was extremely contagious and biblical references that supported the expulsion of lepers from society meant that those diagnosed with leprosy could face social exile. Furthermore, whereas bubonic plague was sometimes interpreted as a sign of communal sin, leprosy in medieval Europe was often interpreted as an indication of individual sin, justifying a leper's isolation. In conformity with these beliefs, the Third Lateran Council (1179) explicitly declared that lepers should be cut off from society and have their own churches and burial places. On the other hand, many authors described leprosy as a gift from God, a trial to test the faith of the afflicted and the charity and compassion of other Christians. As a result, far from being vilified and persecuted, lepers received compassionate support from Church authorities and those who cared for lepers were often viewed as having an aura of sanctity. Indeed, it is significant that archaeologists have found remains with signs of leprosy buried alongside other bodies in local graveyards, suggesting that lepers were not always completely cut off from the community. One highly visible expression of Christian piety toward lepers was the establishment of numerous *leprosaria* throughout Europe for housing lepers. These charitable institutions were frequently located within the precincts of a town or city and provided a place where lepers could receive spiritual and physical care, while minimizing contact and the possibility of spreading the disease to others.

Despite the charitable attitudes, a diagnosis of leprosy could still have profound consequences for individuals in the Middle Ages— social exile. Initially, the determination as to whether a person was leprous, and hence whether the person should face expulsion from the community, fell to local priests or boards of lay officials, leading several physicians to express a concern that cases of leprosy were judged very poorly in their day. The famous Montpellier physician and surgeon, Guy de Chauliac (1298–1368), summarized these views, writing, "Great attention should be paid to the examination and judgment of leprosy, for it is extremely unjust to sequester those who should not be sequestered and to send the infected among the people" (Demaitre 2007, 40). In line with these views, during the thirteenth and fourteenth centuries physicians wrote extensively on how to make an accurate diagnosis of leprosy and distinguish it from other skin disorders, asserting their authority to judge cases of leprosy. Furthermore, although they viewed it as contagious and incurable, physicians still offered extensive advice on treatments to prolong the patient's life and to avoid becoming infected in the first place. Through these efforts, medical men intervened in the process of identifying and treating lepers with the intention of minimizing the social consequences of what was viewed as a frightening disease.

# CHAPTER 7

# Environmental and Occupational Hazards

Environmental and occupational hazards also posed a different range of threats to health in daily life. Authors of the ancient Greek, Ayurvedic, and traditional Chinese medical traditions all asserted the important role played by environmental conditions on individual health. Hippocratic authors warned of the dangers of living in close proximity to swamps, which might be a source of unhealthy miasmatic airs, and the differing influences of the four winds. The author of *Airs, Waters, Places* even indicates that environmental factors accounted for the cultural and physical differences between Greeks and people of other races, like the Scythians. Therefore, the author advises that cities seeking to send out colonies ensure that the new city be built in a salubrious location. Similarly, the *Huangdi Neijing* (*The Yellow Emperor's Classic of Internal Medicine*) considers dietary and health effects on people living in different regions:

> The people of the regions of the East eat fish and crave salt; their living is tranquil and their food delicious. Fish causes people to thirst, and the eating of salt injures the blood. Therefore the people of these regions are all of dark complexion and careless and lax in their principles. Their diseases are ulcers, which are most properly treated with acupuncture by means of a needle of flint. . . .
>
> The North is the region of storing and laying by. The country is hilly and mountainous, there are biting cold winds, frost and ice. The people

of these regions find pleasure in living in this wilderness, and they live on milk products. The extreme cold causes many diseases. These diseases are most fittingly treated with cauterization by burning the dried tinder of the artemisia (moxa). (Veith 1972, 147–148)

In the premodern world, most people lived in rural settings and were usually involved in some form of agricultural labor, facing environmental and occupational hazards particular to these conditions. By contrast, life in cities offered a vastly different experience. Urban dwellers had a greater diversity of occupational opportunities (although requiring a higher degree of specialization) and for this reason villagers from the countryside were often drawn to these centers. However, the confined spaces of cities and the masses of people in them generated new environmental hazards peculiar to urban life.

## LIVING AND WORKING CONDITIONS IN RURAL COMMUNITIES

The vast majority of the population in the premodern world was engaged in agricultural labor. Depending upon the climate and soils, different staple crops were produced: for example, wheat, barley, and millet were grown in northern regions, while rice production was common in the wet regions of Southeast Asia. In some cases, peasant farmers owned and worked their own land (a field large enough to provide for a family, or possibly larger) as freeholders. However, in other cases slaves or serfs (an individual obligated to work the land, but who could not be bought or sold like a slave) worked in the fields held by a wealthy landowner. Serfs were allowed to keep a portion of the produce from the lands they worked for themselves, while delivering the lion's share to their lord, and even freeholders owed taxes or other obligations.

Peasant farmers necessarily made do with minimal possessions. Dwellings were typically small, consisting of no more than one or two rooms. In parts of the world where timber was scarce, people made dwellings out of clay or mud bricks and in northwest China some people lived in artificial caves, digging chambers into the sides of hills. Elsewhere, dwellings were made of wood or bamboo and were likely built to last only one generation before they would disintegrate and be replaced. Such temporary structures often posed threats to inhabitants and many peasants had their homes collapse on them during strong windstorms. In India, evidence suggests that astrologers were often consulted when determining where a house should be built and what layout it should follow (e.g., the door should not face west since that region belonged to the dead). In other parts of the world, such as medieval England, peasant villages followed a haphazard design, and houses were not necessarily placed so as to align with village streets, to be near to water sources, or to minimize or maximize contact with other dwellings. One part of the house would serve as a byre for farm animals and to store farm equipment, meaning that animals and humans lived in very close proximity. Wealthier peasants might be able to afford to build a separate outbuilding to shelter animals, but this was not often the norm. Indeed, the Chinese symbol for "home" is a pictograph of a roof with a pig under it. Hearths for cooking and heat were common and were made of clay or stone where possible, but ventilation was not always adequate and they were also a significant cause of house fires and other injuries. One coroner's report from medieval England relates that a baby died when pigs in the home knocked over its crib and it rolled into the family hearth. In general, a peasant home did not necessarily provide for the safest or most hygienic living conditions.

Rural life and the activities of peasants were typically structured by the agricultural calendar. During the spring months, men would be involved mostly in plowing fields and planting crops, during the late summer months they turned to harvesting, carting, and storing their crops, then in the fall they would be involved in preparing fields for winter crops, butchering animals, and salting or smoking meats. The winter months of December and January, by contrast, were a lull time in terms of agricultural production, but this time was often used to construct and repair fences, homes and outbuildings. All of these activities presented different hazards.[1] The most dangerous time of the year was around the harvest, when men worked long and exhausting hours and might be prone to making careless mistakes. Many men were injured or killed by accidental cuts from the scythes and reaping hooks used to gather the crops, while others were crushed by the heavily laden carts used to carry the harvested crops from the fields, which easily overturned while being drawn across the uneven furrows. The task of storing the loads was also tricky; for example, straw and hay often needed to be stacked in storage barns and it was not uncommon for men to fall from ladders while putting crops into storage lofts at this time of year. In addition to the dangers present at harvest time, farmers were often injured by the large animals they raised for food, or employed in the fields to pull plows or carts.

Women frequently assisted men in the fields, especially during harvest time, and were thus exposed to the same kinds of occupational hazards. For the most part, however, women were injured while engaging in daily activities closer to home, suggesting that this was their chief sphere of work. Although it may seem strange today, one of the most dangerous tasks was drawing water from wells and ponds for drinking, cooking, and washing; the earth around these water sources was often slippery and many women slipped and drowned in them. Women were also commonly injured while preparing the family meals; cooking, baking, and brewing required women to work around large open hearths and carry large vats of boiling liquids. Milking cows, doing laundry, and gathering firewood presented further dangers to women engaged in routine household work. In sum, although women's work was not always as dangerous as men's, we must recognize that they engaged in far more dangerous activities than simply spinning and weaving.

In general, agricultural production existed at little more than a subsistence level for most peasants. They would typically supplement the meager amount of food grown in their fields by raising livestock (chickens, geese, pigs, sheep, etc.) growing vegetables or fruit in home gardens, hunting and fishing, or gathering nuts, herbs, and wild fruits. However, even in the best of times the margin between survival and starvation was thin and in these conditions natural disasters could easily lead to ruin. Farmers along the Nile River in Egypt relied on the predictable flood season to renew the soils and irrigate the crops in their lands, allowing for abundant harvests, hence Egypt's reputation as the breadbasket of the ancient Mediterranean world. The reliable and life-giving floods of the Nile aside, swarms of locusts or other pests, hail, excessive rains and flooding, or droughts could destroy an entire harvest and lead to widespread famine. Years of farming the same fields could also lead to soil depletion, when necessary nutrients were gradually leeched from the ground, so that once fertile lands were no longer as productive as they once had been. Furthermore, marauding armies would often burn fields or steal the little food peasants had stored to feed the soldiers as they passed through an area, not to mention the fact that invading armies would burn villages and slay any peasants they found in an effort to wreak destruction on their enemy's territories. These unpredictable conditions meant that peasants often lived in a chronic state of instability; the lack of food reserves and the inadequate means for transporting supplies to stricken regions meant that famine was an almost endemic scourge in the premodern world. In France between 970 and 1100 C.E., there were no less than sixty years of famine, England reported terrible famines from 1086 to 1125 C.E. and poor harvests lead to famine and privation throughout Europe for much of the fourteenth century C.E., coinciding with frequent plague epidemics. Likewise, China witnessed a series of poor harvests in the seventh century C.E. (brought on by floods and plagues of locusts) and, the fourteenth century was also troubled by a series of widespread famines that coincided with the spread of epidemic disease.

Chinese emperors in the Tang dynasty (618–907 C.E.) regularly assumed responsibility for natural disasters and the government created a series of granaries in strategic locations throughout the empire from which food could be distributed in the event of natural disasters. Not all governments were as prepared to assist starving peasants in times of disaster and in most cases people were left to fend for themselves. Under such difficult circumstances, villagers might turn to eating their seed supplies, set aside for the next season's planting, which would only compound the problem by diminishing future harvests. Stories relate that peasants facing starvation turned to eating grass roots and tree leaves, while some may even have resorted to cannibalism. In other cases, peasants might abandon their villages and move into towns in search of employment and the hope for a better life.

Mining was another of the important rural occupations in the premodern world. People mined for metal ores (gold, silver, copper, iron, red lead, mercury, etc.) as well as precious and semi-precious stones (diamonds, rubies, topazes, sapphires, emeralds, and a variety of crystals). Mines were often operated as a government monopoly, where the state (or an administering official) would claim the proceeds of the mine. Labor in the mines was dangerous. In addition to accidents, miners faced a variety of health hazards including lung diseases from breathing in too much dusty air, exposure to toxic levels of lead (from working in lead and silver mines), or arsenic poisoning (from working with copper ores or arsenic). Lucretius (ca. 99–ca. 55 B.C.E.), a Roman poet and philosopher, commented on working conditions and the noxious airs produced by mines:

> And where there is mining for veins of gold and silver
> Which men will dig for deep down in the earth
> What stenches arise, as the Scaptensula [a mining town in Thrace]!
> How deadly are the exhalations of gold mines!
> You can see the ill effects in the miners' complexions.
> Have you not heard and seen how short is the life
> Of a miner compelled to remain at this terrible task?
> All these exhalations come from the earth and are breathed forth into the
> open light of day. (Nriagu 1983, 110)

Labor in mines was so hazardous that it was often consigned to slaves and criminals, especially in the Greek and Roman worlds. In other parts of the world miners were paid laborers, but not necessarily paid well, and mutinies among miners were not uncommon. As new technologies were invented, such as devices to pump water out of deep mine shafts, mines progressed from being open pit to underground operations, which only compounded the dangers faced by miners, who could be trapped by tunnel cave-ins.

## LIVING AND WORKING CONDITIONS IN URBAN CENTERS

Cities and towns in the premodern world were not large by modern standards. The largest capital cities of the ancient world may have had populations exceeding a half-million inhabitants. Estimates suggest that by the end of the first century B.C.E. Rome and the city of Alexandria in Egypt each had populations of about one million people; the Chinese capital city of Hangchow had a population in excess of one million when Marco Polo visited it toward the end of the thirteenth century C.E. By contrast, Paris, the largest city of medieval Europe had a population of perhaps ninety or one hundred thousand in the fourteenth century. A city with a population of ten thousand or more inhabitants would have been considered large and most towns had a population of no more than around two or three thousand people. Throughout the premodern period the population of towns and cities was not self-sustaining. Deaths brought on by incidences of epidemic disease and general living conditions served continually to whittle down a town's inhabitants. In these circumstances, urban centers required a regular influx of new inhabitants from the countryside to maintain or expand their populations.

### Waste and Sewage Removal

One of the most pressing problems faced by any city is the removal of sewage and other waste. The Romans built a complex network of sewers in their cities to help with waste removal and they were flushed by the water, which overflowed from public fountains fed by a system of aqueducts. Although these sewers were remarkable by comparison to other premodern cities, they were not without their own dangers. Indeed, when the Tiber River flooded, it would often back up into sewers and thence into peoples' homes, and it was not unheard of for a buildup of sewer gases to cause explosions. Latrines connected to sewers also served as an entry point for criminals into the home. Not all homes had latrines served by sewers, however, and most people were likely to use chamber pots, which they would empty into the open streets, despite laws against this practice in many towns. Indeed, the satirist Juvenal (d. early second century c.e.) commented that simply going out to dinner in Rome was dangerous because one risked as many deaths as there were windows to pass under! Much of the waste thrown into streets was washed away by the overflow from public fountains, but more likely the water and sewage were churned together into the ground by the passage of humans, animals, and carts so that the streets were filled with mud and excrement—indeed, several Roman authors commented upon the muddy and filthy condition of Roman streets. Furthermore, the bodies of dead animals and the offal produced by butchers' shops could not easily be removed through the sewers and might be left to decompose in the streets. Although families were expected to pay for the burial or cremation of deceased family members, it was not uncommon to find dead bodies rotting in the streets, if comments by some Roman authors are to be trusted. Authorities might hire workers to clean out cesspits that were not serviced by the network of sewers and to remove dead bodies (human and animal) and other waste (at least from major roadways) to open pits outside the city, but this was not typical.

In the Chinese city of Hangchow in the thirteenth century c.e., public authorities hired street cleaners and paid to have garbage carried by boats that traversed the network of canals to a designated wasteland outside the city. In Hangchow, the wealthy had private cesspits near their homes and would pay to have them emptied when necessary. Most people, however, made do with "horse buckets," which would be left outside their homes and collected by scavengers or nightsoil collectors, commonly called "the pourers," who would sell the contents as manure for gardens around the city. As in other towns, however, it is probable that much of the waste found its way into streets and canals.

Not all cities developed the efficient means of waste removal found in Rome and Hangchow. Indeed, most medieval European cities had an open ditch through the center of main streets that people could empty nightsoil and other waste into, but these channels would often become clogged and municipal authorities did not always pay for workers to keep them clear. Cesspits with privies located in yards or cellars were also typical, and individuals would need to pay to have them cleaned out and the waste carted away every couple of years—in many cases, excrement collected from cesspits was simply dumped into the river (e.g., the Thames River served as the main dumping ground for

London sewage and other waste for centuries). Latrines could often be dangerous places, and numerous reports indicate that children and even adults fell into cesspits and drowned. Tenants in upper stories of buildings might not wish to go to the trouble of descending stairs in the middle of the night to use a latrine, such as one servant in the city of London who "rose naked from his bed and stood at a window of the solar 30 ft. high to relieve himself towards the High Street," and fell to his death (Hanawalt 1993, 29). Although urban leaders passed laws to regulate the placement of latrines, these laws were irregularly enforced and authorities likely only became involved in questions of sewage removal in extreme cases. For example, at an Assize of Nuisances in London in 1347, two men were brought to trial for piping their waste into a neighbor's cellar—the neighbor had not become aware of this until his cellar was overflowing! The city itself must have smelled awful for this homeowner to have failed to notice the smell coming from his own cellar.

In addition to sewage, other waste could quickly accumulate in city streets. Butchers would throw offal from their shops into the streets—one estimate suggests that some 250,000 head of livestock were slaughtered per year in Paris during the thirteenth century—that might collect along with the bodies of dead animals and overflowing sewage channels to putrefy in the sun. The tanning industry, which used urine, tannic acids, lime, and other chemicals in the tanning process, also produced extensive pollution that was washed into streets and nearby streams. The brewers and ale makers, among others, regularly complained about the corruption of fresh water sources (from which water was used for drinking and to make ale). Many towns passed regulations mandating where the butchers and tanners dumped their wastes, or confining them to the outskirts of town, but they were not always enforced. It is little wonder that one sixteenth-century traveler remarked that he could smell the city of Paris two days before he could see it on the horizon!

### Fresh Water and the Risk of Lead Poisoning

Providing fresh water to urban inhabitants presented another range of difficulties. Natural springs and dug wells might provide fresh water for a number of inhabitants, but the quickly growing populations of cities required that additional water be brought in from elsewhere. Once again, Roman engineers excelled in this realm, building vast aqueducts to bring fresh water into cities from great distances. Other cities maintained nearby reservoirs or lakes from which they could draw fresh water. Hangchow, for example, created a nearby artificial lake known as the "Six Wells" and jealously guarded its purity. During the years 1265–1274 the court brought charges against two high officials, who had built houses on stilts over the lake where they washed their hair and did their laundry, charging that "in this way the wines offered up in libation to Heaven and Earth and to the Imperial Ancestors cannot have the required purity. Moreover, the townspeople, who drink no other water but this, run the risk of epidemics" (Wright 1962, 45). Not all towns were as careful about where they drew their water supply, however; for example, many inhabitants of London received water drawn from the Thames River downstream from where the city dumped sewage until the mid-nineteenth century.

In addition to the risk of piping in contaminated water, the pipes themselves may have posed a danger to the drinking water. The pipes were made of different materials, including earthenware (as in Hangchow), wood (as in Basel in 1266), or even lead. Vitruvius Pollio (ca. 50–26 B.C.E.), a Roman architect and military engineer, composed a treatise, *De Architectura*, in which he described the way in which water was delivered to Rome. Concerning the materials used to make pipes, he noted, "Water is much more wholesome when delivered in earthenware pipes than it is when lead pipes are used, for it seems to be made injurious by lead, because white lead is produced by it and this is said to be harmful to the human body" (Cruse 2004, 81). Despite his advice, lead was easier to work with and relatively cheap, so it was widely used in the Roman world for water pipes, as well as for kitchenware and vessels for storing wine and other liquids. The widespread use of lead pipes may have caused increased cases of lead poisoning among inhabitants who drank water supplied by them.

Lead pipes were not the only possible source for lead poisoning. In fact, Romans regularly imbibed a syrup called *sapa*, which was produced by simmering unfermented grape juice in lead vessels and contained a high concentration of lead. *Sapa* was known for being an effective preservative as well as for adding an appealing color, fragrance and sweet taste to wines and it was also added to many foods to sweeten them. Debate continues among scholars concerning the extent to which lead poisoning among the Roman aristocracy contributed to the fall of the Roman Empire. Nonetheless, even if rates of lead poisoning were not high enough to reduce the fertility of the Roman aristocracy as dangerously as some have suggested, it seems clear that many in the Roman world were exposed to far higher levels of lead than would have been healthy. Furthermore, in addition to the risk of lead poisoning from contaminated food and drink, workers who used lead in industries such as painting, plumbing, roofing, sculpture, pewter ware, shipbuilding, enameling, and glazing pottery would have regularly risked occupational exposure.

### The Risk of Fire

Fire was an ever-present danger for residents of premodern cities. The homes of wealthier urban residents may have been larger, with walls around them and slightly wider streets to allow some space and privacy from neighbors, but the majority of buildings in premodern cities were made of wood (or other flammable materials such as bamboo), multistoried, and crowded around a twisting network of narrow streets and alleyways. To gain extra room in upper stories, some buildings had projections that hung out over the street, further narrowing the distance between them and giving an even more claustrophobic feel at the street level (although some cities, like London, passed ordinances stating that projections had to start high enough up from street level to allow a man riding on a horse to pass under them). In a world where everyone had to cook over open flames and used candles or oil lamps to provide light, it is not surprising that fires were extremely frequent and once started they could quickly spread, causing enormous destruction. In addition to cooking fires, blacksmith shops were often cited as the source of blazes, as were scholars who stayed up late at night, reading by candlelight.

The great fire of 64 c.e. in the city of Rome raged for six days and by the time it was extinguished ten of Rome's fourteen districts had been severely damaged, three of which were completely leveled. Tacitus (56–117 c.e.), a contemporary historian who witnessed the fire, reports that following the fire the emperor Nero (r. 54–68 c.e.) mandated that homes be more spaced out and built of brick to help prevent the spread of future fires. During the years of the Roman Republic, Rome had no fire brigade, but Marcus Crassus (ca. 115–53 b.c.e.), who would later be a member of the First Triumvirate with Julius Caesar and Pompey Magnus, notoriously made a large part of his vast fortune by creating a for-hire fire-fighting force. When he learned that a house was on fire he would rush to the location and offer to purchase the home and surrounding buildings for an outrageously low price; if the owners agreed to the sale he would have his men extinguish the fire, but if not he would leave it to burn—a true fire sale! Later, the emperor Augustus (r. 27 b.c.e.–14 c.e.) established a force of about 7,000 watchmen (called *vigiles*), who were given buckets, ladders, axes, and other fire-fighting equipment and required to patrol the city at night looking for fires.

The city of Hangchow in China saw numerous fires in the twelfth and thirteenth centuries, sometimes with several large fires noted for the same year. After two major fires (one in 1132 and another in 1137), which destroyed 13,000 and 10,000 houses respectively, the court erected a series of watchtowers in the most overcrowded districts and manned them with a brigade equipped with fire fighting tools. This brigade would watch for smoke and signs of fire and then use a series of flags and lanterns to indicate the location of the fire so that fire fighters from other towers could join them to help extinguish it. Furthermore, they would patrol the city at night and exact fines on anyone who had fires burning in their homes after lawful hours. Although these measures undoubtedly helped, they could not eliminate the risk of fire, and in 1208 another great fire spread through the city, this one destroying 58,097 homes along a three-mile corridor. Wary of these dangers merchants in Hangchow opted to construct warehouses for their goods in districts that were surrounded on all sides by canals that could work as natural fire breaks, or provide a handy source of water to extinguish any fires.

Although some cities like Rome and Hangchow did develop official fire fighting forces, most cities continued to rely on citizens to watch for fire and organize unofficial bucket brigades. One monk described the spread of a fire in Canterbury in 1174, noting that it started in one house and while the citizens gathered to fight it, a violent wind quickly spread sparks and cinders to neighboring houses setting them alight too. Some of the sparks and cinders landed on the church roof and got between the joints of the lead tiles (lead was sometimes used in roofing in part since it was fire resistant, as opposed to thatch or wooden roofs) until it caught the underlying wooden frame on fire. The account continues:

> Then the people and the monks assemble in haste, they draw water, they brandish their hatchets, they run up the stairs, full of eagerness to save the church, already, alas, beyond help. When they reach the roof and perceive the black smoke and scorching flames that pervade it throughout, they abandon the attempt in despair, and thinking only of their own safety, make all haste to descend. . . .
>
> And now the people ran to the ornaments of the church, and began to tear down the *pallia* and curtains, some that they might save, some to steal them. The reliquary chests were thrown down from the high beam and thus broken, and their contents scattered; but the monks collected them and carefully preserved them against the fire. . . .
>
> Not only was the choir consumed in the fire, but also the infirmary, with the chapel of Saint Mary, and several other offices in the court. (Gies and Gies 2002, 166–167)

In addition to highlighting the bravery of the citizen fire fighters, this author also makes clear the fact that fires were also invitations for looting for some citizens. Indeed, merchants might have had cause to fear the volunteer firefighters as much as the fire!

### Violence and Crime

Premodern cities never had a police force in the modern sense, dedicated to preventing crimes or investigating crimes that had been committed. Many cities did employ night watchmen, however, who were charged with patrolling the streets at night to enforce the curfew. For example, the Gold Bird Guards patrolled in the capital cities during the Tang dynasty in China and maintained a watch post with guards at every intersection. These watchmen would provide a show of force to deter riots and mob violence and they would be involved in apprehending criminals perceived as a threat to the state, but they were not otherwise charged with investigating crimes or apprehending criminals. Rather, private citizens needed to see to their own protection and capture any thief, murderer, or other criminal and take him before a magistrate themselves.

In Rome, homeowners were allowed to kill any thief that broke into their home at night, but if the thief broke in during the day they were expected to raise an alarm and apprehend him with the assistance of neighbors. Similar rules existed in most cities and suggest that neighbors worked together to patrol and protect their own streets. In some cases the townsfolk could act as a mob and captured criminals might be torn apart before they could be delivered to any magistrate. At other times, however, neighborhood watches were not especially effective. One story from India relates that a tradesman awoke at night to find a thief fleeing his shop and dashed into the streets crying, "Stop thief!" The neighbors rushed out with torches to help pursue him. The thief, however, ran through the street's sewage canal, something no upper class Hindu would have dreamt of doing, and then he fled through a graveyard, considered a haunted spot that no one ever dared visit at night. His pursuers, deciding not to risk defiling themselves allowed him to escape. For this reason, wealthy citizens often hired personal guards to provide for their own personal protection and the protection of their shops.

In addition to individual crimes, many cities witnessed a high level of gang violence. In the Byzantine Empire's capital city of Constantinople, for example, youths divided into *demes* or associations, which were linked to the different factional chariot racing teams, denoted by the color of their uniforms: Blues, Reds, Greens, and Whites. Political factions in the city often tried to manipulate these gangs to their own ends so that they were not only social but also political associations. As a result, these gangs were often involved in hooliganism and causing riots in the city. The most famous riot occurred in 532, when people gathered at the Hippodrome to watch the races and the Blues and Greens joined forces crying out "Nika" (meaning "conquer") and started to assault the palace with the intention of overthrowing the emperor, Justinian I (r. 527–565), with the support of various senators. After five days of rioting, Justinian sent word (along with bags of gold) to the Blues, reminding them that he had always supported their faction and pointing out that the new emperor they hoped to install was a Green. After this, the Blues broke off their alliance with the Greens and ceased to riot and Justinian sent his armies in to kill and dispel the remaining rebels—about thirty thousand rioters were reported killed.

In other cities, guilds provided the primary social unit by which people identified themselves. In medieval Europe, it was common for rivalries to develop between youth gangs from different guilds. Apprentices from one guild would sometimes band together and make forays into neighborhoods of rival guilds to start fights and many of these apprentice gangs engaged in prearranged mock battles that often ended in severe injuries or even deaths. Gangs of male youths were also known to attack and rape vulnerable women. Students were perhaps the most notorious of all youths, widely condemned for the violence and mayhem they caused in cities. In many European universities, students were expected to enter clerical orders, signified by the tonsure or the shaving of the crown of the head. Clerical status conveyed important privileges in medieval society, including protecting the individual as sacrosanct—any violence perpetrated against someone with clerical status was punished with immediate excommunication. Furthermore, clerics were not subject to civil law, but rather to the canon law of ecclesiastical courts, which often gave lighter punishments for crimes than civil courts (the most extreme punishment was to be stripped of one's clerical status, whereas the death penalty was common for a variety of offenses under civil law). Together these privileges allowed students a great margin for causing trouble without the expectation of serious retribution. In Paris at the beginning of the thirteenth century, for example, students were known for provoking brawls in taverns with guild apprentices, relying upon their clerical status to protect them from any response and with the knowledge that they would face a lighter punishment than the lay youths for their actions. No wonder that King Philip Augustus

(r. 1180–1223) marveled at the bravery of students who waded into fights carrying swords, but not wearing any armor or helmets—their shaved heads advertising their clerical status were armor enough!

## NOTE

1. Barbara A. Hanawalt, *The Ties That Bound: Peasant Families in Medieval England* (Oxford: Oxford University Press, 1986) offers extensive insight into the hazards faced by agricultural laborers. She examines records produced after coroners' inquests into cases of accidental deaths in medieval England to learn about the daily lives of peasants. Although she focuses on medieval England, her findings about the occupational hazards faced by agricultural laborers are likely similar to conditions in other pre-modern agrarian communities.

# CHAPTER 8

# Surgery and Manual Operations

Humans have been performing a variety of surgical operations and physical manipulations on the body for a very long time. Archaeologists have discovered evidence that Neolithic humans were performing trephinations, carving holes into the cranium, as early as 10,000 B.C.E., and the indication of new bone growth along the cut edges of the skull indicate that the individuals who underwent such operations had a high survival rate. Indeed, many skulls have been trepanned more than once. Today, trephination is used to relieve pressure on the brain caused by internal bleeding from head wounds, for example. While it is not clear why these operations were performed among prehistoric peoples, they may have been performed for religious as well as medical reasons, perhaps to release malign spirits from the head or as a form of ritual mutilation, similar to cutting off joints from fingers as is done in some primitive societies (e.g., to placate ghosts or honor the recently dead). In any event, the practice indicates the extent to which prehistoric peoples developed and employed surgical techniques.

As remarkable as the practice of trephination might seem, it was likely an elective procedure and prehistoric peoples probably needed to treat injuries such as fractures and dislocations far more often. Archaeologists have discovered bones from the Neolithic period with healed fractures, indicating that prehistoric peoples could also treat broken bones. Indeed, they may have used some kind of splint, as is done among many primitive tribes today, using tree branches or even soft clay that hardens into a protective cast around the injury. It is not inconceivable that prehistoric tribes also employed various means for reducing dislocations; indeed, primitive societies today often treat dislocations through massage or employ more active manipulations to alleviate these conditions.

Although we have no evidence for how prehistoric man dealt with lacerations and other kinds of open wounds, it is likely that they employed techniques similar to those seen used in primitive tribes today. Anthropologists have found that some primitive peoples employ a variety of means for staunching the flow of blood, for example using herbs or roots, often with astringent or antibacterial qualities, that they apply to the wound in the form of powders or poultices. In other cases, they also apply heat, in the form of hot stones or needles, or even the direct application of fire, to staunch blood flow. Suturing wounds with stitches was likely rare among prehistoric peoples and they were probably left open during treatment. Premodern tribes in different parts of the world today, however, display several other methods for closing wounds, which may have been employed in some early societies. For example, some tribes in South America and in parts of India have used large ants to close wounds; the edges of the wound would be brought together and grasped in the ant's mandibles, after which the ant's body would be removed, and the jaws, stiffening in death, would remain to hold the wound closed. Another means of suturing is employed among the Masai in Africa, who use a long acacia thorn, which is struck through both open edges and then the ends are united and twined together, drawing the wound closed. In the absence of suturing, however, a variety of substances might have been used as wound dressings (including animal substances, such as milk, fat, and even excrement) to keep the wound covered and aid in healing. It is therefore likely that through the empirical process of trial-and-error, our prehistoric forebears developed a number of methods of wound treatment.

In the early civilizations we examine, surgeons were predominantly concerned with treating fractures and wounds. However, as surgeons became more adept at healing injuries they also expanded their skills to treat other physical conditions through surgery, including bladder stones, cataracts, and hernias. In some cases, surgeons even developed techniques for cosmetic surgery. As the theories and activities of healers became increasingly complex and specialized, those who focused on curing diseases and internal disorders (physicians or doctors) were distinguished from those who treated external conditions or provided physical treatments (surgeons). In this chapter we will examine the activities and status of the surgeon in different cultures.

## SURGERY IN ANCIENT MESOPOTAMIA

There are very few references in medical texts from ancient Mesopotamia to surgical activities or treatments suggesting that this knowledge was learned through apprenticeship and practice rather than through reading texts. The Code of Hammurabi, however, does offer some insight into surgical practice. It consists of 282 laws, which enumerate a range of regulations and prescribe punishments for various crimes, inscribed in the cuneiform script on a roughly seven-foot-tall, black diorite stone dating to about 1750 B.C.E. While it says nothing about the use of drugs or other treatments for internal diseases, it does include several regulations stipulating the *asu*'s fee for various procedures and, thus, giving a sense of the range of surgical operations he might be called upon to perform.

> 215: If a physician performed a major operation on a seignior with a bronze lancet and has saved the seignior's life, or he opened up the eye-socket of a seignior with a bronze lancet and has saved the seignior's eye, he shall receive ten shekels of silver.
>
> 216: If it was a member of the commonalty, he shall receive five shekels.
>
> 217: If it was a seignior's slave, the owner of the slave shall give two shekels of silver to the physician.
>
> 221: If a physician has a set a seignior's broken bone, or has healed a sprained tendon, the patient shall give five shekels of silver to the physician.
>
> 222: If it was a member of the commonalty, he shall give three shekels of silver.
>
> 223: If it was a seignior's slave, the owner of the slave shall give two shekels of silver to the physician.

Furthermore, punishments for unsuccessful cures or medical malpractice are also recorded.

> 218: If a physician performed a major operation on a seignior with a bronze lancet and has caused the seignior's death, or he opened up the eye-socket of a seignior and has destroyed the seignior's eye, they shall cut off his hand.
>
> 219: If a physician performed a major operation on a commoner's slave with a bronze lancet and has caused (his) death, he shall make good slave for slave.

220: If he opened up his eye-socket with a bronze lancet and has destroyed his eye he shall pay one-half his value in silver. (Meek 1969, 175–176)

Clearly, the risks were great for the *asu*, but so were the rewards—it would take a carpenter 450 working days to earn ten shekels!

In specifically medical texts we find a few more detailed references to treating wounds with the bronze knife. In most cases they refer to using the knife to make incisions to release pus from abscesses or boils. For example, one text, "Prescriptions for Diseases of the Head," describes a typical procedure:

If the ailment mentioned above is painless, and the very surface of the flesh is intact; if, when you open, pus squirts out and keeps flowing: the name of this disease is "little she-fly." If the wind has blown onto the patient, it is a case of Pabil-sag [the god]: you can operate [on] it. To remove it, attack this disease with the point of the knife. After cutting it open grind boiled plaster, salt of ammonia and powder of [unknown mineral]. Apply all this onto the diseased surface and make a dressing of it. If the disease has reached into the bone, cut all around, scrape and remove. (Majno 1975, 52)

As this passage makes clear, the Mesopotamian *asu* learned how to make wound dressings to wrap and protect injuries. Surviving texts describe a few examples of the ointments or salves that could be made to wash and cover the wound, along with recommendations for how often to change bandages, but there is no specific mention of suturing wounds in the medical texts.

Other surgical procedures might have been performed by different kinds of practitioners. The code refers to the *asu alpim u lu imerim* ("physician of an ox or an ass," a veterinary surgeon), specifying the fee he could receive for performing a major operation on an animal to save its life and also the fine the veterinary surgeon would pay if his operation caused its death. It is likely that castration was one of the tasks the *asu alpim u lu imerim* might perform on animals, and other documents indicate that humans were also castrated, either as a form of punishment or because many court employees were expected to be eunuchs. The code also recognizes the *gallabu* (barber), who would perform minor manual operations. In the law codes, the *gallabu* is associated with branding or cutting the mark of the owner onto slaves, but some scholars have suggested that he might also perform other kinds of minor surgery such as extracting teeth, a function carried out by barbers in other early civilizations. Whether or not the *gallabu* was responsible for doing dental operations, we know that this was one of the kinds of surgical procedures regularly performed in ancient Meso-potamia. Dental problems were often associated with larger medical concerns and tooth extraction was regarded as the necessary treatment, as can be seen in this letter from an *asu* to the king:

> Replying to what the king my lord wrote me, "send me your true diagnosis." I have given my diagnosis to the king my lord in one word: "Inflammation!" He whose head, hands, and feet are inflamed, owes his state to his teeth: his teeth should be extracted. On this account his insides are inflamed. The pain will presently subside; the condition will be mostly satisfactory. (Sigerist 1951, 435)

This interesting passage suggests that the *asu* might try to cure some internal disorders through physical operations, but it is unclear whether he would perform the extractions himself, or leave this to another specialist.

## SURGERY IN ANCIENT EGYPT

The medical papyri reveal a good deal about the surgical abilities of the *swnw* and the kinds of instruments they might employ. In most cases, the surgical operations described in the papyri are for treating traumas or lancing abscesses, but otherwise surgery was fairly limited in scope. No uniquely surgical instruments have been found from the period of the pharaohs, reinforcing the impression that the ancient Egyptians did not conduct difficult surgeries that might require specialized equipment. Most of our information about Egyptian surgery comes from the forty-eight surgical cases described in the Edwin Smith papyrus, which appears to have been aimed at teaching.

Dislocations and fractures are among the most prevalent conditions described in the Edwin Smith papyrus. The *swnw* is advised on how to reduce dislocations of the shoulder and the jaw, and on how to reduce fractures so that broken bones could be set. Case 35 provides an elaborately detailed description of how to reduce a fractured clavicle:

> If you should examine a man having a break in his collar-bone, and you should find his collar-bone short and separated from its fellow. You should say concerning him: "One having a break in his collar-bone, an ailment which I will treat." You should place him prostrate on his back, with something folded between his two shoulder-blades; you should spread out with his two shoulders in order to stretch apart his collar-bone until that break falls into its place. You should make for him two

splints of linen, and you should apply one of them both on the inside
of his upper arm and the other on the under side of his upper arm. You
should bind it with *ymrw*, and treat it afterward with honey every day,
until he recovers. (Breasted 1930, 350–352)

An analysis of six thousand bodies buried in cemeteries in Aswan
from 4000 B.C.E. to 500 C.E., found two hundred with united fractures. Although some revealed perfect alignment of the bones, most
instances were less successful and several display excessive shorten-
ing of the limb and misalignment of the bones, revealing how difficult
it was to sustain the traction necessary to maintain alignment (Jones
1908, 455–458). The accounts of treating fractures suggest the use of
bandages, but also of some form of splint as described for the clavicle
fracture, to hold the bones in place while they healed.

Bites and stings from a variety of creatures, including snakes, scorpions, lions, crocodiles, and humans, defined the other major category
of traumas sustained by ancient Egyptians. The first concern for snake
and scorpion bites was whether the person might expect to survive
the venom, depending upon what kind of snake bit him. Treatment
included using a combination of magical incantations and surgical
remedies. One papyrus offers this advice, "What is to be done for the
bite of the male snake? Incise his wound/bite with the knife treatment many times. Then you should apply a bandage to it (with) red
natron . . . salt, etc." Or, "Another [remedy] to drive out the swelling.
Incise his wound/bite with the *des*-knife many times on the first day.
Apply salt 1/8 or natron. Bandage the wound with it" (Nunn 1996,
188). The emphasis on swift treatment (numerous applications on the
first day) and the need to cut around the swelling at the wound would
serve to reduce the swelling and possibly to minimize the absorption
of the venom. For bites where there was no concern for venom, treatment mainly consisted of bandaging various drugs over the injury, as
was done with other forms of wounds, and there is no mention of cutting around the site. For example, the doctor is told, "If you examine
the bite of a crocodile and you find it [with] his flesh piled up and its
two sides being separated, then you should bandage it with fresh meat
on the first day, likewise all wounds of a man" (Nunn 1996, 190).

The treatment for a crocodile bite is indicative of the approach to
curing all kinds of gaping wounds: bandage with fresh meat on the
first day. Following the initial treatment with fresh meat, the *asu*
might bind other substances (such as honey, grease, and lint) over the
wound. These procedures were likely effective since fresh meat has
been shown to contain coagulants that could help staunch bleeding

and the antibacterial quality of honey would likely serve to reduce the chance of infections and thus accelerate healing.

## SURGERY IN ANCIENT GREECE AND ROME

### Hippocratic Surgeons

The Hippocratic texts reveal that the *iatros* was prepared to perform a wide variety of surgical procedures to treat injuries and wounds. For example, two entire texts, *On Fractures* and *On Joints*, were dedicated to explaining methods for realigning broken bones and reducing dislocations. While two strong men would serve to carry out the procedure in most cases, the texts also discuss the construction of an innovative apparatus that could mechanically draw the limb back into alignment. For example, in order to repair a spinal distortion, the *iatros* is advised to give the patient a warm bath, presumably to help relax the muscles, and then strap him down to a plank, with straps under the armpits and around the hips, so that they could be drawn apart, while the *iatros* massaged the spine back into alignment. If necessary, the author says that a wheel and axle could be attached to either end of the board and to the straps so that they could be turned to stretch the spine; furthermore, he notes, "This reduction apparatus is easy to regulate as regards greater or less force, and has such power that, if one wanted to use such forcible maneuvers for harm and not for healing, it is able to act strongly in this way also" (Withington 1944a, 301). Clearly, the author recognized another potential use for this device and was not thinking of the directive in the Hippocratic *Oath* that the physician should do no harm.

Hippocratic surgery was not limited to the treatment of wounds and injuries, however; indeed, the authors also discussed a number of elective operations. In addition to lancing boils, the knife was used for the surgical removal of nasal polyps, for removing swollen tonsils, and for cutting ulcerated varicose veins. Cautery was also used to treat certain surgical conditions such as hemorrhoids: "Force the anus out as far as possible with your fingers; heat the irons red-hot, and burn until you so dry the hemorrhoids out that you do not need to anoint: burn them off completely, leaving nothing uncauterized" (Potter 1995, 381–383). The *iatros* might also undertake more daring procedures, such as that described in *On Diseases II* for draining pus from the pleural cavity:

> Cut as low as possible so that the pus may flow out more easily. Cut between the ribs, the skin first, using a knife with a rounded blade. Then take a pointed knife, wrap its blade in a cloth so that only the point will

protrude as much as the length of a thumb's nail, and cut through [to the pleural cavity]. Let out as much pus as you think best, then put in a tent of raw linen attached to a thread. Let out the pus once a day. On the tenth day, having removed all the pus, put in a tent of fine linen; then inject warm wine and oil through a small tube, so that the lung, accustomed to be moistened by the pus, may not remain suddenly dry. Remove in the evening the oil and wine injected in the morning; that injected in the evening, remove it on the following morning. When the pus becomes as thin as water, slippery to the finger, and scanty, put into the wound a hollow tin drain. When the pleural cavity becomes dry cut the drain shorter little by little, and allow the incision to heal as you retrieve the drain. Signs that the patient will escape death: if the pus is white and pure and contains streaks of blood, there are good chances of healing. But if pus . . . on the next day flows thick, greenish and fetid the patients die after the pus has run out. (Majno 1975, 157)

Aside from this extreme case, however, most Greek surgery was fairly conservative and fairly limited in scope.

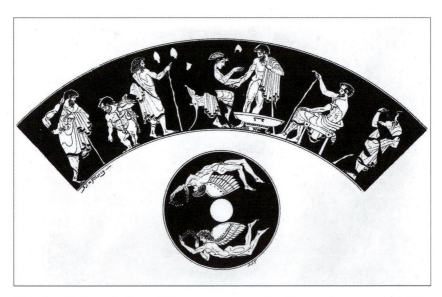

This is a flattened view of the images on a Greek vase from around 480–460 B.C.E. It depicts a doctor letting blood from a patient in the center, while other patients, including a dwarf and an amputee, wait for assistance. Some patients use crutches or walking sticks and have bandages shown on their arms or legs. The small white shapes in the space above the doctor are the cups used for cupping. (Wellcome Library, London)

The Greeks also applied surgery for treating internal disorders. The humoral theory, which explained disease as caused by an imbalance in the body's humors, dictated that treatment should aim at restoring the balance through dietary changes, or by purging the excess harmful humor. One means of removing excess humors was through the application of bloodletting (also referred to as phlebotomy or venesection) and several Hippocratic treatises recommend the use of the knife to let blood from veins. Although some texts merely recommend phlebotomy without specifying a location, others advise that veins be opened in different parts of the body, depending on the condition. For example, *On the Nature of Man* recommends that for pain in the loins and testicles blood should be let from behind the knee or the inner side of the ankle, but in other conditions, it is recommended that blood be let from the inner arm at the elbow. It appears that the application of the knife to let blood for the purposes of treating internal disorders was likely one of the most common surgical procedures performed by the Hippocratic doctors. In a later period, Galen (129–ca. 216 C.E.) wrote no fewer than three treatises dedicated to bloodletting: *On Venesection, On Venesection against Erasistratus* and *On Venesection against the Erasistrateans*. He elaborated upon the Hippocratic theories, making phlebotomy not only the preferred treatment for a wide range of internal disorders, but also the main tool for preventive health. Galen advocated letting blood from different veins in the body, depending upon the location and nature of the internal disorder, and argued that other factors, such as the season and the age of the patient, should also be taken into consideration when determining when and how much blood to let. Following Galen, bloodletting became a fundamental method of treatment throughout the Greco-Roman world and continued to be practiced in the Islamic world and during the European Middle Ages.

Cupping was another manual practice in the Greek world that, like phlebotomy, required physical application on the body to treat internal disorders. Cupping entailed putting a piece of burning material into a little metal cup so that when applied to the skin, the flame would be extinguished and create a vacuum, holding the cup to the skin. These could be applied to the skin to help draw humors to the site, to help rectify localized humoral imbalances in the body. The practice of "wet" cupping (as opposed to "dry" cupping) entailed scarifying the skin to cause bleeding before applying the cup, so that excess humors could be drawn out of the body. This treatment was so closely associated with doctors that the cupping vessel became one of the main symbols of a doctor, very much as the stethoscope might be a symbol of the doctor today.

## Roman Surgeons

Although often suspicious of Greek theoretical medicine, Romans were adept at surgical practice. Archaeological discoveries have revealed that Roman medical practitioners possessed surgical kits with a number of specialized surgical tools, including scalpels, probes, hooks, forceps, bone levers, cautery needles, cupping vessels, trephining saws, and rectal or vaginal specula. Indeed a surgeon in the town of Rimini from around 257 C.E. possessed a kit with over 150 instruments with many versions of the same instrument each displaying subtle differences. The variations in the instruments suggest that they were adapted for specialized procedures (or perhaps for operating on people of different sizes) and attest to wide range of Roman surgical expertise. Archaeologists have also revealed false teeth (made with both real and artificial teeth) and a variety of artificial limbs attesting to the Roman ability to make prosthetic devices.

Although he was not a practicing doctor himself, the Roman author, Aulus Cornelius Celsus (ca. 25 B.C.E.–ca. 50 C.E.) offers an excellent account of the extent of Roman surgical practice in the seventh book of his *De Medicina*, where he considers "the third part of the Art of Medicine . . . that which cures by the hand." Celsus holds surgical skill in high regard, declaring that it is more reflective of the doctor's expertise than other forms of treatment since people often recover from diseases as much from luck as from any medicines, whereas it is obvious when the surgeon's actions are the reason for success (Spencer 1961, 295). He reveals that Roman surgeons were more adventurous than their Hippocratic forebears and were willing to attempt many more difficult procedures. These included the surgical removal of cancerous tumors (although he lamented that using corrosive substances to burn them out only made them grow faster, and that cutting them out was often ineffective because they only grew back after scar tissue had formed), hernia repair, removal of bladder stones, and amputation. Celsus also describes in great detail the operation for couching cataracts (moving aside or extracting a lens that has become so cloudy that it blocks light from reaching the retina), which he claims is the most delicate of procedures. The patient should be seated and have his healthy eye covered so he will not see what is about to happen next:

> Thereupon a needle is to be taken pointed enough to penetrate, yet not too fine; and this is to be inserted straight through the two outer tunics [layers of the eye] at a spot intermediate between the pupil of the eye

and the angle adjacent to the temple, away from the middle of the cataract, in such a way that no vein is wounded. The needle should not be, however, entered timidly, for it passes into the empty space and when this is reached even a man of moderate experience cannot be mistaken, for there is then no resistance to pressure. When the spot is reached, the needle is to be sloped against the suffusion itself and should gently rotate there and little by little guide it below the region of the pupil; when the cataract has passed below the pupil it is pressed upon more firmly in order that it may settle below. If it sticks there the cure is accomplished; if it returns to some extent it is to be cut up with the same needle and separated into several pieces, which can be the more easily stowed away singly, and form smaller obstacles to vision. After this the needle is drawn straight out; and soft wool soaked in white of egg is to be put on, and above this something to check inflammation; and then bandages. (Spencer 1961, 345–353)

The range of complex surgical procedures described by Celsus reveals the extent to which surgical expertise had advanced in the Greco-Roman world by his time. Not to diminish the Roman surgeon's skills, we should remember that these operations were carried out without the benefit of anesthetics. Therefore, it should not come as a surprise that when Celsus describes the qualities of an ideal surgeon he recommends that while the surgeons should feel pity for the patient, he should not be "moved by [the patient's] cries, to go too fast, or cut less than is necessary; but he does everything just as if the cries of pain cause him no emotion" (Spencer 1961, 297). Patients must have been suffering indeed, to decide to undergo any form of elective surgery!

## SURGERY IN INDIA

### Surgical Training and Procedures

Early Ayurvedic medical texts, the *Susruta Samhita* in particular, contains several chapters on a variety of surgical procedures. The author of the *Susruta* praises surgery as the oldest and most important of all the branches of the Ayurveda, since "it contains all that can be found in the other branches of the science of medicine as well, with the superior advantages of producing instantaneous effects by means of surgical instruments and appliances" (Bhishagratna 1907, 8). Furthermore, the author maintains that the surgeon, "skilled in the art of using surgical instruments, is always successful in his professional practice, and hence the practice of surgery should be commenced at the very outset of medical studies" (Bhishagratna 1907, 70).

Becoming a successful surgeon, however, was not an easy task. First, the surgeon needed to become familiar with the use of a wide range of instruments, including knives, probes, and implements for cautery; the *Susruta* recommends that young surgeons learn how to use their instruments by practicing on dead animals, gourds, cucumbers, watermelons, or filled water skins. Furthermore, while acknowledging that religious prohibitions against contact with dead bodies posed a difficulty, the author of the *Susruta* maintained that the surgeon should familiarize himself with anatomy by examining a dead body in the following manner:

> The excrementa should be first removed from the entrails and the body should be left to decompose in the water of a solitary and still pool, and securely placed in a cage (so that it may not be eaten away by fish nor drift away), after having covered it entirely with the outer sheaths of *Munja* grass, *Kusa* grass, hemp or with rope etc. After seven days the body would be thoroughly decomposed, when the observer should slowly scrape off the decomposed skin etc. with a whisk made of grass-roots, hair, *Kusa* blade or with a strip of split bamboo and carefully observe with his own eyes all the various different organs, external and internal, beginning with the skin as described before. (Bhishagratna 1911, 172)

Despite this advice it is likely that most surgeons did not acquire much anatomical knowledge beyond what they could learn by treating wounds, however. As a result, the surgeon's basic knowledge of anatomy most likely revolved around learning the locations of the 107 *marmas*, vital parts or seats of life in the body. Injury to any of these sites was supposed to lead to rapid death without judicious treatment and the surgeon needed to carefully avoid damaging these areas when performing operations.

Bloodletting and cautery are perhaps the two most common surgical procedures described in the *Susruta*. Phlebotomy could be accomplished with the knife or with leeches—indeed, in one chapter the author explains the classification, selection and appropriate care of leeches, as well as their application for bloodletting. Cautery could also be accomplished by different means, either with caustic substances or hot-irons. Both of these forms of what we might consider minor surgery might be used to treat an internal disorder (e.g., an imbalance of *doshas* leading to disease), to staunch bleeding, or to treat an external ulcer. Indeed, so far as the author of the *Susruta* was concerned, surgery and internal medicine were closely related and, therefore, the surgeon needed to be familiar with the written tradition of theoretical medicine.

### Early Methods of Reconstructive Surgery

The *Susruta* describes a number of difficult elective surgical procedures, including operations for removing anal fistulas, reducing inguinal hernias, and couching cataracts. Perhaps the most remarkable procedures covered in Indian medical texts are those for plastic surgery. Piercing the earlobes for wearing jewelry as ornamentation and to ward off malign influences was a common practice in ancient India. The piercing procedure and post-operative treatment are portrayed in the text along with advice on how to cope with complications caused by profuse bleeding or infection (including the risk of tetanus). Once pierced, the earlobes were gradually stretched over time by carrying heavy ornaments and in some cases, whether by the weight or in the course of an argument, the earring would tear through the lobe. This condition appears to have occurred regularly enough to merit extensive coverage in the *Susruta*. Indeed, the author classifies no fewer than fifteen varieties of tears and ten different diseases that affect torn earlobes!

In response to these conditions, Indian surgeons developed methods of reconstructive surgery to repair the torn lobes. Taking the type of tear (e.g., whether the ends of the bifurcated lobes were of equal size, thick or shriveled, short or extended, etc.) into consideration, the surgeon would scarify the two parts of the torn lobe and wash the bleeding ends with different substances, depending upon which of the *doshas* was deemed to be disordered. Then the surgeon would adhere the two ends, anoint them with honey and clarified butter, wrap them in cotton, tie them together with string, and leave them to heal (with continued application of medicines and appropriate attention to diet and regimen). If all went well, the two ends of the lobe would grow together over time, but the *Susruta* offers advice on what to do should further complications arise. Thus, we find a pioneering account of plastic or reconstructive surgery from the ancient world.

The *Susruta* also describes an even more difficult technique for rhinoplasty, replacing noses cut off in battle or, more often, as a common form of punishment for adultery. A flap of skin would be cut from the patient's forehead, leaving a strip attached at the bridge of the nose. The flap would then be twisted down and sewn over the scarified skin around the hole on the face, with two tubes inserted to help mold the nostrils. The strip of skin at the top of the nose would provide nourishment through blood vessels, until the scarified tissue of the flap and around the hole grew together and produced new blood vessels. The ability to carry out this procedure successfully would be very valuable, as the author notes, since "the physician, who is well conversant with these matters, can be alone entrusted with the medical treatment of a king" (Bhishagratna 1907, 154). Essentially the same procedure is still used today.

### Surgery and the *Vaidya*

The *Susruta* is certainly remarkable for its detailed description of several elaborate surgical procedures and for the effort to unite the practice of surgery with the theoretical concepts of Ayurvedic medicine. It is, however, unlikely that the surgical activities described continued to be practiced by the *vaidyas* (doctors) much beyond the time when the *Susruta* was composed. Later Ayurvedic medical texts do not reflect any further development of surgical techniques and those that do cover surgery are mainly based on sections copied from the *Susruta*. Historians believe that as the caste system developed during the first millennium CE, taboos against cutting into the body may have led *vaidyas*, trained in the Sanskrit literary tradition and coming from the upper social castes, to avoid the practice of surgery. The result was that surgery gradually ceased to be represented in the written tradition of Ayurvedic medicine as *vaidyas* focused their attention on internal medicine.

There is evidence, however, that the surgical practices discussed in the *Susruta* were continued by members of lower social castes, who functioned as barber-surgeons. These barber-surgeons would not have been trained in the learned, written tradition of Ayurveda; rather, they would have learned and passed on their surgical skills via apprenticeship. The argument in favor of the continuation of surgery outside the literary tradition is supported by the example of the famous rhinoplasty operation witnessed by British army surgeons in India in 1793. A Maratha named Cowasjee, who had been a bullock-driver with the British army, had been captured by the forces of the Tipu sultan and had his nose and hand cut off. In the following year, he and his associates who had suffered the same fate, sought the aid of a man from the brick-maker's caste near Poona, who performed the reconstructive surgery. The British surgeons, thoroughly impressed by this operation, wrote up a description of it, along with diagrams and an engraved illustration, for publication in Europe. The fact that the procedure was performed by a member of the brick-maker's caste, who probably knew no Sanskrit, strongly suggests that the techniques first recorded in the *Susruta* persisted outside the written medical tradition.

## CHINESE SURGERY

### The Low Status of Surgery and Surgeons

Little written evidence exists concerning the practice of surgery in ancient China. Within traditional Chinese medicine, even skin disorders and wounds were treated according to the theory of systematic correspondence and as a result the medical literature contains few references to any kind of surgical procedures. It may be too simplistic to blame the Confucian dogma against opening the body for the apparent lack of attention to surgery, but in any event, it does appear that surgical skill was not highly regarded and the surgeon was considered inferior to the physician. As a result, surgery existed outside the learned tradition of Chinese medicine and, therefore, was typically practiced by illiterates, who learned their technical skills through apprenticeship and were unfamiliar with the theoretical, written medical tradition.

The written tradition of Chinese medicine does celebrate the possibly legendary activities of one learned surgeon, Hua Tuo (110–207 c.e.). He is said to have traveled widely in China, learning from popular medical traditions wherever he went, and to have served as physician to kings. Among other things, Hua Tuo is recognized for his advocacy of acupuncture and physical exercise as remedies, but he was most famous for his surgical skills. One famous story attributes to him the discovery of an anesthetic known as *mafeisan*, a powder dissolved in a fermented beverage, which he used on a patient on whom he performed some form of abdominal surgery. Another legend relates that Cao Cao, ruler of the Cao Wei kingdom in northern China, requested Hua Tuo's presence at court, but the physician refused to attend him. Infuriated, Cao Cao had Hua Tuo imprisoned and sentenced for execution. While in prison prior to his execution, Hua Tuo wrote down his medical learning, but when he could not smuggle it out of prison he had it burned. Another legend relates that a few pages were snatched from the flames, containing his explanation for the procedure of castration, but otherwise all of his medical learning, including the recipe for *mafeisan*, was lost!

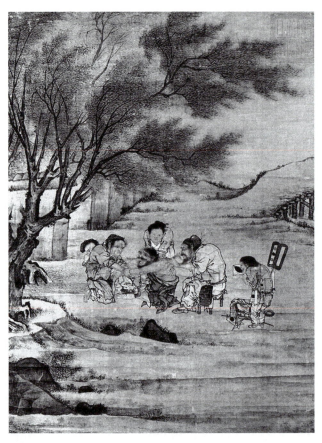

In this painting by Li Tang (1049–1130) a Chinese village doctor is shown applying moxibustion to a patient, who is shouting with pain while being held still by another man. (Takeyoshi Tanuma/Time Life Pictures/Getty Images)

### Moxibustion and Acupuncture

Although the practice of surgery was not highly regarded in ancient China, the application of acupuncture, which was a physical operation, became a highly valued therapeutic practice favored by physicians. The origin of acupuncture is not clear, but it seems to have developed out of early surgical activities. The earliest Chinese medical texts discovered in the Mawangdui gravesites, which date to about 168 B.C.E., do not mention acupuncture, but they offer insight into the development of theories that would later support the practice. These texts describe a series of eleven *mai* (vessels) running through the body and emphasize that disease arises from disturbances in the flow of *qi* (vapor) through them. The therapeutic practice advocated for treating disorders is cauterization by means of applying burning materials on the body along the path of the affected *mai* in order to influence the movement of *qi*. This form of cauterization soon developed into the practice of moxibustion, the specific use of mugwort tinder (moxa) to cause the burn. The practice of bloodletting may also have provided a precursor to the use of acupuncture. The Mawangdui texts do not mention bloodletting (although it is discussed in the *Huangdi Neijing*), but they do discuss the use of lancing stones to open abscesses. Furthermore, those texts indicate that the *mai* contain both *qi* and blood and the congruence between blood vessels and *mai* is suggestive. The *Huangdi Neijing* recommends bloodletting to release bad blood and to stimulate the flow of *qi*. In this regard, the practice of bloodletting may also have contributed to the development of acupuncture therapy.

It is clear, however, that by the first century BCE acupuncture was adopted as a supplement to moxibustion as the primary means of correcting the flow of *qi* in the body. The *Huangdi Neijing* provides an elaborate explanation of the procedure, although it does not always clearly distinguish between the use of moxibustion or acupuncture. This text identifies twelve channels or meridians in the body through which *qi* flows and identifies 365 specific points on the body along these channels for applying moxibustion or acupuncture. According to the theoretical system, the body was in a constant flux between a state of *shi* (fullness) and *xu* (emptiness), and acupuncture could be used to either deplete or drain off fullness or stimulate the flow of *qi* to combat emptiness. Unlike bloodletting, therefore, acupuncture was used either to remove excesses and sedate the body or to correct deficiencies and to tonify the body. Indeed, as it developed acupuncture became a bloodless form of surgery—any bleeding from the needlepoint would represent a lapse in technique. The acupuncturist needed to consider a number of factors when applying the needles, as one passage in the *Huangdi Neijing* makes clear:

> The nine needles are of different size, shape, and use. When acupuncturing excess, one must sedate. Insert the needles and await the arrival of *yin qi*. When one feels a cooling sensation under the needle, remove the needles. In deficiency, one must tonify. After needle insertion, await the arrival of *yang qi*. When there is a warming sensation, remove the needles. Once you grasp the *qi* with the needle, be very attentive and listen so as not to lose the opportunity to manipulate the effects. Treat disease according to where it is located; determine whether to insert deeply or shallowly. When the disease is located deep, insert deeply. When the disease is superficial, needle shallowly. Although there is a difference

in depth of penetration, the principle of awaiting the *qi* is the same. (Ni 1995, 192–193)

Later texts, including the *Nanjing* and Huangfu Mi's (215–282 C.E.) *Zhenjiu Jiayijing* (*The ABC of Acupuncture and Moxibustion*), provide more detailed descriptions of the use of needles applied to specific points to restore health and more fully relate the use of acupuncture to the paradigm of systematic correspondence that forms the theoretical basis of traditional Chinese medicine. Over time, the number of points identified for acupuncture rose. Finally, during the Song dynasty (960–1279 C.E.), Wang Weiyi (ca. 987–1067) produced two bronze statues of a man into which 657 holes were drilled representing acupuncture points, which could be used for teaching. These models were filled with water and then covered with wax and students would be expected to practice their acupuncture skills, knowing that if they hit water they had found the proper acupuncture point. Wang Weiyi also compiled the *Tongren Shuxue Zhen Jiu Tujing* (*Illustrated Manual of the Bronze Man Showing Acupuncture and Moxibustion Points*), as a guide to teaching for those who did not have access to the bronze models.

## SURGERY IN THE ISLAMIC WORLD

Arabic medical literature from the tenth and eleventh centuries provides extensive coverage of surgery. These texts draw extensively upon the Greek and Roman written tradition and as a result, Islamic books on surgery cover many of the same procedures without additions or emendations. Despite the lively medical literature, some question remains concerning the extent to which the written works on surgery reflected actual surgical practice in the Islamic world. In several surgical writings, physicians described a surgical procedure, but then commented that they did not know anyone who actually performed the operation, or indicated that they themselves chose not to do it. Indeed, it is suggestive that although the famous physician, Abu Bakr Muhammad ibn Zakariya al-Razi (d. ca. 925, known as Rhazes in the Latin West), described 900 case histories from his own practice in his formal medical texts, he did not discuss performing any surgical procedures aside from bloodletting and cauterization.

One explanation for the lack of innovation or indication of personal experience in surgical writings may be attributed to the fact that Arabic literature recognized distinct medical specialties and a division of labor, whereby physicians did not undertake surgery themselves. One physician noted,

As for the handling of these matters with surgery, that is a function of some of the assistants to the physician. The same is true for bloodletting, cautery, and phlebotomy . . . All these are functions of the physician's attendants. As for the physician, he should be concerned with treating the patient by means of diet and medicaments and he should not include manual techniques [that is, surgery]. (Pormann and Savage-Smith 2007, 122)

Indeed, by the fourteenth century, Arabic authors recognized a number of specialized medical practitioners apart from physicians, who focused on particular manual operations, including oculists, circumcisers, phlebotomists, cuppers, bone-setters, cauterisers, and those who administered enemas. These practitioners would have a lower status than the physicians, trained in the written medical tradition, and they likely developed their own skills through apprenticeship and practice.

## Abu al-Qasim al-Zahrawi

Not all physicians eschewed surgical practice, however. Abu al-Qasim al-Zahrawi (fl. ca. 1000, known as Albucasis in the Latin West) was one of the physicians who earned a reputation for his surgical skills in Islamic Spain. Although he often expresses caution about undertaking surgical procedures and does not suggest many innovative surgical techniques in his encyclopedic work, *The Arrangement of Medical Knowledge for One Who Is Not Able to Compile a Book for Himself*, al-Zahrawi does describe eighteen surgical case histories from his own practice. Eleven of the cases were for the treatment of wounds (from arrows, spears, and knives), four involved the removal of tumors or growths, two were cases where he chose not to operate (including a man who amputated his own foot and hand), and for the final case he provides no details about treatment. His texts make it clear that despite his status as a physician, al-Zahrawi did not hesitate to perform surgical treatments himself. For example,

My own experience was this: a slave-girl seized a knife and buried it in her throat and cut part of the trachea; and I was called to attend her. I found her bellowing like a sacrifice that has had its throat cut. So I laid the wound bare and found that only a little hemorrhage had come from it; and I assured myself that neither the jugular vein nor an artery had been cut, but air passed out through the wound. So I hurriedly sutured the wound and dressed it until healed. And no ill befell the maid except for a hoarseness in the voice, but nothing more; and after some days she was restored to the best of health. Hence, we may say that tracheotomy is not dangerous. (Spink and Lewis 1973, 338)

Al-Zahrawi's encyclopedia is remarkable for its inclusion of a number of illustrations of surgical instruments. His surgical chapters describe the use of a number of sophisticated instruments for use in typical surgical procedures. Modifying a procedure for the removal of stones in the duct carrying urine from the bladder, al-Zahrawi describes the use of a fine drill that would be inserted through the urinary passage to break up the stone, as an alternative to the procedure described in Greek sources that required making an incision to remove the obstruction. In another case, he describes using a scissor-like instrument with transverse blades for removing tonsils: the surgeon would hold the tongue with a tongue depressor, grasp the swollen tonsil with a hook, and then cut through the gland with this ingenious instrument. Al-Zahrawi also invented a knife for lancing abscesses, which was designed so as not to alarm the patient. The instrument, which he called the "deceiver," was made by concealing the blade between two curved plates attached to a handle so that it could be extended for use only as needed. The development of such specialized instruments for use in these more common operations makes clear that some Islamic surgeons did continue to advance their craft in this period.

## SURGERY IN THE MEDIEVAL WEST

### Surgeons and Physicians

During the European Middle Ages, surgery flourished as a craft tradition, and surgeons were trained through apprenticeship. Following the rise of universities in the twelfth century, many physicians made a categorical distinction between the *physicus* (physician) trained in the written tradition of learned medicine at the university, and the *chirurgicus* (surgeon), who learned his skills in practice, with little if any exposure to the medical works of the Greek, Roman, and Arabic authors.

The physician claimed expertise in the practice of internal medicine, prescribing drugs to cure the humoral imbalances that caused disease, while the surgeon was expected to limit his practice to the application of manual procedures to treat wounds and external conditions, including skin disorders. Although physicians claimed the prerogative to regulate the practice of phlebotomy, since it was undertaken to treat internal disorders and therefore depended upon the physician's extensive theoretical knowledge, surgeons were the ones who would typically apply the knives and often did so without a physician's supervision. Thus, patients might also turn to surgeons when looking for cures to a variety of internal diseases through bloodletting.

In addition to the professional *chirurgicus* a number of other individuals in medieval society might offer surgical cures. Barber-surgeons would not only offer a shave and a haircut but would also be ready to let blood or pull teeth as part of their regular services—indeed, the barber's bowl could serve both to hold warm water for shaving and to catch blood drained through phlebotomy. Furthermore, a wide range of empirics, who specialized in the treatment of a particular condition, including fractures, bladder stones, cataracts, and hernias, also flourished. Faced with competition from these other practitioners, surgeons often sought to protect their own craft knowledge. For example, after relating his cure for hemorrhoids in his book the English surgeon, John of Arderne (1307–1380 or 1392), advised, "The doctor should be careful in case any of the bystanders see how it is done as the excrescences are opened up. Since once the barbers grasped the method they would usurp this cure for themselves to the considerable shame and harm of the master surgeons" (Jones 1994, 304).

## The Rise of Rational Surgery

From the twelfth to fifteenth centuries there was an explosion of new treatises on the practice of surgery, written in both Latin and vernacular languages by physicians. This explosion was in part fueled by the rapid influx of translations of Arabic and Greek surgical texts into Latin (the writings of al-Zahrawi, known as Albucasis in the West, were especially influential) that provided a theoretical foundation for the practice of surgery. One of the first to write a surgical text was Roger Frugard (before 1140–ca. 1195), a physician and surgeon at Parma, who produced his *Chirurgia* (*Surgery*) around 1170. The *Chirurgia*, which covered the treatment of injuries in a head-to-toe arrangement, became a standard text for Latin instruction in surgery in the universities in Italy and at Montpellier until the late thirteenth century when it was supplanted by newer Latin books on surgery and the direct study of Greek and Arabic texts, especially that of Albucasis.

Frugard's *Chirurgia* helped to spawn a new genre in medical writing in Western Europe, the Latin general surgery. Many of the authors of these new Latin surgical texts self-consciously sought to elevate the study and practice of surgery to the status of a learned science, founded upon abstract rational principles (McVaugh 2006). Two physicians working in Bologna sought to describe surgical practice with reference to the Greco-Arabic surgical texts, the procedures used by their contemporaries and their own practice: Teodorico Borgognoni (ca. 1205–1298), who started writing handbooks on surgery in the 1240s, and Bruno Longoburgo, who produced a his *Cyrurgia magna* (*Great Surgery*) in 1252. Both authors expanded the study of surgery beyond the treatment of wounds to include the treatment of cancers and conditions such as arthritis and gout. Furthermore, their goal was to situate the study of surgery within the learned tradition of medicine, and to consider significant earlier surgical scholarship from authors including Galen, Albucasis, Avicenna, Rhazes, Haly Abbas, and Roger Frugard. Thus, both authors argued that surgery was a subject that should be learned, at least in part, from books. Teodorico expresses this opinion in this way:

> It behooves practitioners of surgery . . . to frequent the places where skilled surgeons operate, and to attend their operations diligently, and to commit them to memory . . . because all things which are necessary to the art cannot be included in books, cannot easily be foreseen, and many of these frequently happen to the operator. . . . [However,] they must needs be well-read, and even if they be aided sometimes by experience, yet frequently will they fall into error and into confusion. I scarcely think that anyone can understand surgery without schooling [in texts]. (Campbell and Colton 1955, 4–5)

Another Italian author of a Latin surgical manual, Guglielmo da Saliceto (1210–1277), who wrote Latin treatises on surgery in the 1270s, went so far as to argue that surgery was a *scientia* ("science," or learned body of knowledge) that could be learned entirely from books, without ever practicing. The new genre of Latin rational surgical manuals was spread to France at the end of the thirteenth century by Lanfranc (d. 1315), a student of Guglielmo da Saliceto, who fled Italy to go first to Lyon and then to Paris, and Henri de Mondeville (ca. 1260–ca. 1320), a pupil of Teodorico Borgognoni, who taught at Montpellier and Paris. Both physicians composed surgical manuals in Latin and like their predecessors they based their identities as surgeons on their knowledge of the learned textual tradition and clearly hoped to see the teaching of surgery institutionalized within the universities as a theoretical subject alongside the study of medicine.

The last of the great medieval authors of a Latin surgical manual, Guy de Chauliac (1298–1368) wrote his massive *Inventarium sive Chirurgia Magna* (*The Inventarium or Great Surgery*) around 1363. Guy earned his degree in medicine at Montpellier and studied surgery in Bologna before beginning his own medical practice and spent most of his career serving as physician to three different popes in Avignon. Although he addressed his work to surgeons, Guy appears to have been less concerned than his predecessors with strictly defending the rationality of surgery. He did not hesitate to relate cases where he had learned procedures from empirics and readily discussed the importance of his own training through practice. Nonetheless, the *Inventarium* surveyed the principle textual authorities and the historical development of the rational study of surgery to his day and provided a comprehensive, systematic overview of the discipline and as such marks the culmination of the medieval tradition of rational surgery.

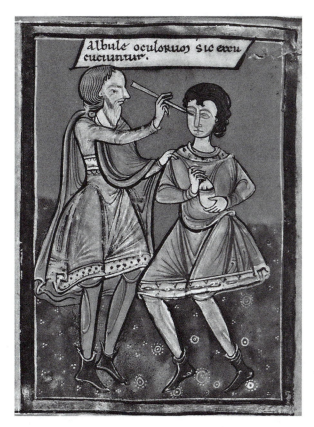

This is an illustration from an early fourteenth-century copy of Roger Frugard's manual on surgery, which depicts the procedure for couching a cataract. The long needle would be inserted into the eye to dislodge the clouded lens. (The British Library/StockphotoPro)

## Vernacular Surgery Texts and Craft Practice

In their effort to promote surgery as a rational, textual subject worthy of being taught in the universities, many authors of Latin surgical manuals were dismissive of the activities of craft surgeons and de-emphasized the value of empirical learning. For example, drawing a distinction between those surgeons trained through apprenticeship and the new rational surgeons, Henri de Mondeville emphasized that "a surgery that is learned only by practice and that is carried out lacking any prior theoretical instruction, like the surgery of peasants and illiterates, is a purely mechanical effort, neither theoretical in a proper sense nor a proper science or art" (McVaugh 2006, 61). Guy de Chauliac, by contrast, sought out opportunities to observe the practice of craft surgeons and report on their successful cures. Indeed, increasingly in the fourteenth century learned surgeons appear to have yielded the practice of dangerous invasive procedures to the empirical specialists. In particular, the rational surgeons increasingly avoided operating for cataracts, hernias and bladder stones, leaving those procedures to a variety of traveling craft operators, who were not necessarily familiar with the written tradition of surgery. The learned physician-surgeons would have had a good reason for doing this—as Henri de Mondeville complained when noting the difficulties faced by surgeons, "the surgeon has to perform manual operations, and any mistake in his treatment leaps to the eye or touch and is bound to be set down to him; but mistakes made by physicians are not obvious to the senses and can be ascribed to 'nature' or 'the governing force of the body'" (McVaugh 2001, 332). In this regard, it might have been more advantageous for the physician-surgeon to have prescribed drugs and other treatments for cataracts and other conditions and left the manual operations to the lower-status empirics.

Nor is it possible to believe that empiric surgeons of the later Middle Ages were unaware of the tradition of rational surgery. Indeed, during this period the proliferation of translations of surgical manuals into vernacular languages (spoken languages of the people: French, German, and English among others), including Guy de Chauliac's *Inventarium*, meant that many more people had access to the rational surgeries. Likewise, during this period original works on surgery were also being produced in vernacular languages. The production of so many surgical manuals in the vernacular attests to the increasing demand for technical books on surgery and a growing community of surgeons who were literate in vernacular languages, if not in Latin.

# CHAPTER 9

# The Brain and Mental Disorders

The concept of psychiatry did not exist until the nineteenth century, and premodern views of psychopathology do not easily coincide with our own. Mental disorders or conditions that caused an individual to appear as though they were not in control of their own faculties, or in their "right mind," posed a particular challenge for premodern societies. Conditions causing psychoses, delusions, and fits were not always viewed as belonging in the sphere of the doctor, but rather were thought to be brought on by divine or supernatural powers, and thus more properly falling under the control of priests. When viewed from this perspective, it was not necessary to offer a physiological explanation for the onset of the symptoms. Medical authors, however, were often interested in the relation between the physical body and the way in which it influenced behavior and the expression of emotions, impaired the faculties of cognition, or inhibited voluntary control over one's action. They looked for theoretical explanations for mental disorders that would conform to their own understanding of the body and disease and that would dictate a rational therapeutic response. Neither group gained a monopoly over the treatment of such conditions and as a result, responses to mental illness in early civilizations combined both religious and medical efforts.

## THE MIND AND ILLNESS IN MESOPOTAMIA
## AND EGYPT

There is no evidence that the Mesopotamians or the Egyptians associated the brain with memory, intelligence, or emotions. Indeed, in the process of embalming, the brain was the only major organ the Egyptians removed and discarded, suggesting that they did not view it as significant. Emotions and the mind seem, rather, to have been associated with the heart in both cultures. The Egyptians specifically linked the faculties of the mind with the *ib* ("heart," sometimes also translated as "mind"), the seat of consciousness. For example, the Ebers papyrus connects the *ib* with memory, noting that "as to [when] his *ib* [mind] is drowned: this means that his *ib* is forgetful like one who is thinking of something else" (Ghalioungui 1963, 129).

The Mesopotamians used a number of different terms to describe conditions that we might associate with epilepsy, but which they also linked to a variety of mental disorders. Furthermore, it is not clear from their terminology whether the terms distinguished between different conditions or were used to speak of the same condition. The Akkadian word, *bennu*, for example, is used to describe the following symptoms: "If a man is quivering all the time when lying down, shouts like the shouting of a goat, roars, is apprehensive, shouts a lot all the time, (then it is) the Hand of *bennu*, the demon deputy of (the moon-god) Sîn" (Stol 1993, 6). The Sumerian term, *miqit samê* ("what has fallen from heaven"), refers to similar symptoms: "If a sick man's neck turns to the right, time and again, while his hands and feet are paralyzed, his eyes are now closed, now rolling, saliva flows in/from his mouth, he makes . . . sounds" (Stol 1993, 8). These terms are often used interchangeably (along with terms like *miqtu*, "hand of god or goddess" and others) to denote conditions, whether epileptic or not, associated with spasms and falling down. Other phrases used to denote the same symptoms are associated with conditions that seem to verge on madness, such as "Spawn of (the god) Sulpaea":

> If a seizure seizes him at sunset and, as it seizes him, a wailing voice shouts to him and he himself responds every time, (if) he time and again shouts: "my father, my mother, my brothers, my sisters, (are) dead,". . . and stops (shouting) every time,. . . after having cried he falls asleep and does not get up: (if), as the seizure leaves him he does not know that he has cried: [he is suffering from] "Spawn of Sulpaea"; it will not go away. You burn him with fire in his illness. (Stol 1993, 15)

This example reveals that these conditions are not clearly linked with what we might consider epilepsy, but rather reflect a range of possible mental illnesses. While "hand of god" (sometimes "hand of goddess") is often associated with seizures, it sometimes also has other symptoms so that the sufferer, "curses the gods, he speaks insolence, he hits whom(ever) he sees," or "he has [?] of heart-break, time and again, and forgets his (own) words, time and again" (Stol 1993, 25). Thus, this array of symptoms variously associated with seizures and linked by a number of, often interchangeable, terms appear to indicate some understanding of mental illness.

Those suffering from these various conditions were viewed in a negative light within Mesopotamian society. The Code of Hammurabi specifically mentions the condition *bennu* (possibly epilepsy) indicating that it was viewed as detrimental in slaves: "if a seignior purchased a male (or) female slave and when his month was not yet complete, *bennu* attacked him, he shall return (him) to his seller and the purchaser shall get back the money which he paid out" (Meek 1969, 177). The birth of a child having epileptic-like seizures was also viewed as an ill omen and as we have seen, those with Spawn of Sulpaea deemed incurable might be burned, or in some cases buried alive. Indeed, common curses such "may a bad *bennu* fall upon you," or wishing that your enemies might suffer "a *miqtu* that does not go away," are also indicative of the social reaction to these kinds of conditions.

## MENTAL HEALTH AND HUMORAL MEDICINE IN ANCIENT GREECE AND ROME

The Hippocratic author of *On the Sacred Disease* specifically considered the problem of epilepsy. As in the Mesopotamian world, epilepsy was viewed as a disease caused by divine powers in the early Greek world, but the Hippocratic author argued that epilepsy and all mental disorders had naturalistic causes that could be explained in terms of an imbalance in the body's humoral physiology.

> Madness comes from its [the brain's] moisture [caused by excess phlegm]. When the brain is abnormally moist, of necessity it moves, and when it moves neither sight nor hearing are still, but we see or hear now one thing and now another, and the tongue speaks in accordance with the things seen and heard on any occasion. But all the time the brain is still a man is intelligent.
>
> The corruption of the brain is caused not only by phlegm but by bile. You may distinguish them thus. Those who are mad through phlegm are quiet, and neither shout nor make a disturbance; those maddened through bile are noisy, evil-doers, and restless, always doing something inopportune. These are the causes of continued madness. (Jones 1923, 175–177)

This position meant that mental health could be explained in the same terms as physical health and that mental illnesses could be treated by the same methods used to treat other diseases, namely with diet, regimen, drugs, and phlebotomy.

Greek natural philosophers and medical authors also offered theories about the ways in which race and gender might influence an individual's mental state and personality. In another Hippocratic text, *Airs, Waters, Places*, mental dispositions are explained in terms of the environmental and seasonal influences on a population. For example, the author argues that the different climates in Europe and Asia are largely responsible for the physical form of the inhabitants as well as their personal character; the mild and uniform seasons of Asia makes the men weaker, while the dramatic seasonal changes in Europe make men there stronger: "For the frequent shocks to the mind impart wildness, destroying tameness and gentleness. For this reason, I think, Europeans are also more courageous than Asiatics. For uniformity engenders slackness, while variation fosters endurance in both body and soul; rest and slackness are food for cowardice, endurance and exertion for bravery" (Jones 1984, 133). In this sense, a people's mental dispositions were shaped by their complexion (or individual balance of humors) and also by the influence of external factors on individual development. Slightly later, Aristotle (384–322 B.C.E.) would argue similarly that the female of the species tends to be dominated by the quality of cold whereas the male is dominated by the quality of heat. He maintained that these qualitative differences, beyond the humoral complexion, incline women to being timid and slow-witted (traits associated with the quality of coldness), whereas men were brave, outgoing and intelligent (traits associated with the quality of heat). Galen of Pergamum (129–ca. 216 C.E.) further refined these thoughts about the role of humoral physiology in determining an individual's mental dispositions and in explaining mental illness, offering a more systematic consideration than his predecessors of the ways in which an individual's humoral and qualitative composition would shape both body features and character traits.

## THE MIND AND MENTAL HEALTH IN AYURVEDIC MEDICINE

The ancient Hindu scriptures contain several descriptions of characters suffering from mental illness—stories of madmen (*unmattaka*). The *Ramayana*, for example, relates the story of Lord Rama and his family, many of whom suffered from what we might define as depression; his grandfather was depressive after the death of his wife and eventually starved himself to death, and his father suffered bouts of depression after accidentally killing a blind man and later when he was separated from his children, from which condition he eventually died. Lord Rama himself suffered from depression while searching for his abducted wife, Sita, becoming despondent, pensive and forgetful, crying out in anguish, fainting, and experiencing loss of appetite, before finally committing suicide. Similarly, in the *Mahabharata* the protagonist, Arjun, suffers from depression when he realizes that he will have to kill his relatives in battle, experiencing a dry mouth, unsteady thoughts, and wet palms. He is eventually alleviated of his symptoms after being counseled by Lord Krishna.

The Ayurvedic texts also consider mental health from the perspective of medical theory. These texts located the *manas* (mind) and the *citta* (consciousness) in the heart; they are responsible for directing the senses and controlling cognition. By contrast the eternal *atman* (self/ soul), which is shaped by the *karman* ("deeds," good or bad actions from previous lives), is only conscious by virtue of its connection with the senses. In order to maintain health, the individual needs to balance the needs of body, mind, and soul. Mental illnesses can arise from a number of physiological factors, including the blockage or destruction of pathways from the heart which convey the *manas* and disruption of the *doshas*, brought on by an inappropriate diet, or sudden mental shocks from extreme emotions. On the other hand, the medical texts also allow that mental illness could arise from the wrath of the gods or demonic possession.

The observations about the relationship between the mind and body led the authors of Ayurvedic medical texts to develop notions of individual personality types shaped by their *prakriti* (personal temperament) or the preponderance of the different *doshas* in their body at the time of generation. The *Susruta Samhita* describes seven personality types according to which *dosha* (or combination of *doshas*) was predominant at birth. A person of the *vata* temperament (having a preponderance of *vata*), for example, is impulsive, restless and prone to wakefulness, while a person with a *kapha* temperament is known for self-control and unselfishness. Individuals from the different temperamental types can be recognized by their distinct bodily features, reflecting the close association between mind and body; in the *Susruta* we learn that a person of the *vata* personality is distinguished by his unshapely body, rapid movement and shifty eyes, while the *kapha* type often has curly hair and well-proportioned limbs.

Vagbhata's *Astangahrdaya* (*The Heart of Medicine*), written around 600 C.E., brings together many of the theories about mental illness from the early Ayurvedic tradition. He identifies six categories of *unmada* (insanity or madness) with natural causes; insanity caused by derangement of one of the three *doshas* (*vata, pitta,* or *kapha*), as an effect of another disease, by the anxiety from facing an unbearable loss, or as an effect of poison (including the effects of alcohol). These conditions are likened to epilepsy, which the medical texts indicate should be treated with the same methods used for those suffering from *unmada*. Patients would initially be treated with purgatives or enemas to clear the blocked pathways along which the *manas* flows. One such potion called for cooking cow's urine with ghee and some other herbs and spices, which the author declared to be "the best thing for banishing insanity, demons, and epilepsy" (Wujastyk 2003, 247). Other remedies called for making pastes and ointments that could be applied to the eyes or nasal passages, as well as burning various substances as fumigants to restore the appropriate equilibrium of the *doshas*. Vagbhata also suggests treatment through different forms of what we might call shock therapy, including flogging the patient and then throwing him into a dark pit or room, covering her with mustard oil and then tying her down stretched out in the sun, or having police grab him and threaten him with corporal punishment in the name of the king! In cases where *unmada* was caused by demonic possession, Vagbhata suggested similar cures, but noted that they should be supplemented with various rituals and prayers to appease the demons, depending upon the nature of the demon causing the illness.

## MENTAL ILLNESS IN TRADITIONAL CHINESE MEDICINE

Chinese literature and folklore offers useful insight into how people viewed mental illnesses in traditional China. Legends of the wandering holy man Daoji (d. 1209) highlight the ways in which he transgressed the rules of his own Buddhist religious tradition, earning him the appellation of "Crazy Ji" and leading to his removal from a monastic community. A later account of the life of Daoji relates:

> Crazy Ji's original name was Daoji. He was wild and did not pay attention to small details of conduct. He used to drink wine, eat meat [in violation of monastic dietary rules against drinking wine and eating meat], and drift about the marketplace. People thought he was mad, for which reason they called him "Crazy Ji." (Shahar 1998, 50)

In another account we learn, "Crazy Ji was getting wilder and wilder; often he would go to the Cool-Spring Pavilion and turn somersaults in it, falling flat on the ground. He would enter the Summoning-the-Monkey Cave and invite the monkey to somersault with him; or else, he would lead a group of children to the wine shop, where he would sing mountain songs" (Shahar 1998, 61). His madness, expressed as nonconformity and religious eccentricity, was viewed as a marker of his piety and members of the laity revered him as a saint and spread stories about his remarkable healing powers. Daoji is just one among many "crazy monks" (*dian seng*) or "mad monks" (*feng heshang*) described in Chinese literature. These monks were generally recognized for their unusual behavior, including breaking religious rules, wearing rags that barely covered their bodies, having irregular speech, behaving erratically, and eating strange things. Despite their wildness, the laity often revered these wandering monks, who were separated from the monastic establishment, as holy fools and miracle workers. The stories largely reflect an undercurrent of lay hostility toward the Buddhist monastic establishment, but at the same time, they offer a perspective on Chinese beliefs about madness. In these contexts, no stigma was attached to those who displayed the symptoms of what we might recognize as mental illness.

Another folkloric tradition in China suggests a widespread popular belief in the supernatural or demonic origin of mental disease. Malign fox demons were particularly common culprits in causing mental disorders, going back at least to the period of the Han dynasty (206 B.C.E.–220 C.E.). One story from the late eighth century C.E. tells of a well-mannered ten-year-old boy, who was suddenly struck by an illness that completely transformed his personality. The father summoned a Taoist healer who, declaring that "this boy suffers from a sickness which is caused by a fox demon," brought about a cure and then cautioned that henceforth he would need to treat the boy every day to maintain his health, to which the father agreed. The story continues:

> Though the boy was cured of that disease, still he lacked a sufficient quantity of soul, wherefore he uttered every now and then insane talk, and had fits of laughter and wailing, which they could not suppress. At each call of the doctor, the father requested him to attend to this matter too, but the other said: "This boy's vital spirits are kept bound by a specter, and are as yet not restored to him; but in less than ten days he will become quite calm; there is, I am happy to say, no reason to feel concerned about him." And the father believed it. (Veith 1963, 148)

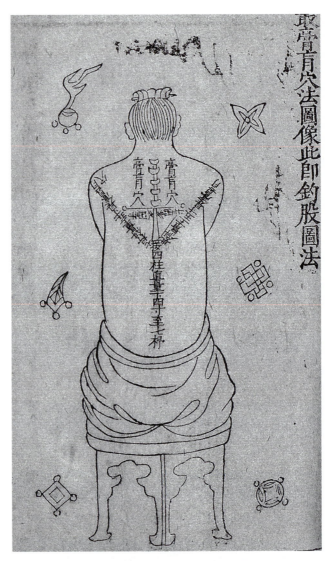

This is a woodcut illustration from a copy of the *Tongren Shuxue Zhen Jiu Tujing* (*Illustrated Manual of the Bronze Man Showing Acupuncture and Moxibustion Points*) by Wang Weiyi, published in 1443. The image depicts the method for locating the vital points for acupuncture. The point of intersection in the middle of the back was considered a panacea against a variety of conditions, including madness and memory loss. (Wellcome Library, London)

Nonetheless, the boy continued to suffer from this condition and the father called in another doctor and then a third. These three doctors began to fight and the father, rushing back into the sick room, found three foxes on the ground, panting and exhausted, and realized that they were the three doctors, who had first caused and then tried to prolong the disease in a scheme to get his money. In his anger, he beat the foxes to death and thereafter the boy no longer suffered from his mental affliction. Beliefs like those expressed in this story about the demonic or supernatural cause of madness portrayed the sufferer as an innocent victim of an outside force, and attached no stigma to the individual afflicted with mental illness, although it is likely that a burden of shame fell on the family of the patient in traditional China. Treating mental illness caused by angry ghosts, demons, or other supernatural beings often required some form of exorcism. This entailed rituals of curative magic, which were sometimes associated with violence, including beating patients and exposing them to cold and uncomfortable living conditions to drive the supernatural beings from their bodies.

Traditional Chinese medicine does not clearly distinguish between psychological and physiological conditions and there was no specialized branch of medical theory devoted to psychiatric medicine. This does not mean that Chinese medicine did not recognize psychiatric disorders—indeed, the aforementioned accounts from Chinese literature and folklore shows that they did—but mental illnesses were not formally set apart from somatic disorders in the textual medical tradition as they were in other cultures. Medical authorities spoke of seven emotions (joy, anger, grief, worry, fear, desire, and fright) and the need to regulate them by avoiding displays of excess emotion for the sake of maintaining health. Furthermore, the internal organs are linked to different emotions: for example, the heart with the emotion of joy, the kidneys with fear, the liver with anger, the lungs with grief, and the spleen with worry. Excessive emotions could harm the organs and lead to derangement of the flow of *qi* in the body and thus to disease, or conversely, diseases of the internal organs could engender excessive emotions. As a result, psychological and emotional disturbances were viewed as important symptoms of physiological illnesses, not necessarily as independent mental disorders.

The *Huangdi Neijing*, however, does discuss two major types of madness brought on by a *yin-yang* imbalance: *dian* (an overabundance of *yin*) and *kuang* (an overabundance of *yang*). A patient with the *kuang* form of madness is described as manifesting the following symptoms:

He will discard his clothes and run about, mount heights and sing, or get to the point of not eating for several days. He will leap walls and ascend rooftops. In short, all the places he mounts are beyond his ordinary abilities . . . he will talk and curse wildly, not sparing relatives or strangers. Not wishing to eat, he will run about wildly. (Chiu 1981, 75)

The *kuang* form of madness, therefore, is associated with an excited and agitated state in which the patient is in constant motion and displays misanthropic tendencies. By contrast, the *Nanjing* (*Classic of Difficult Issues*) describes those with the *dian* form of madness as being passive, apathetic, and even staring blankly in a catatonic state. Later medical authors related these conditions to seasonal and other environmental causes. Sun Simiao (581–682), for example, pointed to a pathogenic (disease-causing) *feng* (wind): "When *feng* enters the cardinal conduit of *yang* polarity, *kuang* ensues; when *feng* enters the cardinal conduit of *yin* polarity, *dian* ensues" (Ng 1990, 36).

Physicians who considered *kuang* and *dian* predominantly advocated treating them with the same therapies they would use for somatic diseases, namely with drugs and acupuncture. Some physicians, however, felt that these cures were sometimes insufficient for relieving emotional or mental disorders. Zhu Zhenheng (1281–1358), who believed that *dian* and *kuang* were caused by excessive emotions, proposed countering those emotions with their opposites so as to neutralize the excess and cure the madness; for example, a person suffering from pathogenic (disease-causing) joy would be encouraged to feel anger or worry. The physician Chang Ts'ung-cheng (1156–1228) was perhaps even more famous for his unorthodox methods of treating madness. In one case, he was called in to treat a woman who had frequent violent screaming fits and on whom drugs had been ineffective. He had two of her female assistants dress in outlandish clothes and sent them to the patient, who burst into laughter for the first time in months; on the following day he sent them to the patient dressed as animals, again inducing laughter; on the third day he had them wolf down a huge feast in front of the woman, which led the patient to recover her own appetite for food. In another form of shock therapy, he had a person with a mental illness tied to a large wheel and had assistants spin it until the patient vomited a greenish fluid and finally asked to be let down, after which he was cured! The naturalistic cures offered by physicians indicate their belief that mental disorders were not caused by supernatural forces, but in some cases of shock therapy the cures resemble the kinds of cures offered by religious healers seeking to exorcise the possessing fox demons. Perhaps the patients (or their families) had more faith in these more dramatic forms of treatment for mental illnesses.

## MENTAL ILLNESS IN ISLAMIC MEDICINE

The Arabic word *majnun* ("possessed" or "madman") was the most commonly used designation in early Islamic society for an individual who would be described as "mentally ill" today. Labeling an individual as *majnun* was usually a social decision, and physicians had only a small role in making the diagnosis. Islamic literature, such as the collection of tales in *The Thousand and One Nights*, portrays some cases of madness as positive conditions from which the sufferer would not wish to be cured. In particular, those whose madness was inspired by God, such as the wise fool or holy fool, who speak the truth and dedicate their lives to serving God despite the risks, might be revered as holy mystics, so people believed that: "The madman knows best his own soul. True discourse must be heard from a madman" (Dols 1992, 349). Indeed, the Prophet Muhammad was often accused of being a madman for his willingness to speak the truth. On the other hand, under the law the insane were viewed as having the same legal status as children, unable to have independent control over their own decisions or to own property and thus requiring legal guardians who would see to their protection. Therefore, being labeled as *majnun* was not always positive.

Spirits known as *djinn* were frequently mentioned in the Quran as causing madness in humans by possessing an individual's body and driving him mad—thus the term *majnun* means both "possessed" and "madman." Such possession could be thwarted by Prophetic and religious healers and by prayer. One text prescribes the use of magical talismans, prayers, and massage for those with epilepsy, apoplexy, and hysterical fits, so that

the devil should be massaged out from the important organs to the less important ones and eventually out of the body through the lower extremities. The massage develops in most cases to violent beatings, which may be carried out with the hand, with a stick, show or even with a holy object, like the wooden shoe of the Madjthub.

It is easier to drive out devils when the bodily condition of the possessed person is at the lowest. It is a common belief that the *djinn* prefer well-built, corpulent patients. This explains why the patients are fed so badly. Neglect of cleanliness leads to the same result. (Dols 1992, 237)

The medical authors followed their Greek forebears in offering naturalistic explanations for the causes of mental illnesses. Ibn Sina (d. 1037, known as Avicenna in the Latin West) dismissed the belief that djinn caused melancholia in his *Canon of Medicine*, saying, "If it were caused by the djinn, it happens by changing the temperament to black bile, for melancholia's cause is the dominance of black bile. Thus, the cause of that black bile may be djinn or something else" (Dols 1992, 81). While not denying the possibility of a supernatural cause for melancholia, he sought to frame it in terms of humoral physiology and thus made clear that mental illnesses would be amenable to cures by natural medicines.

Although many Islamic medical authors discussed the diagnosis and treatment of mental disorders, Ibn Sina's *Canon of Medicine* came to be viewed as the most authoritative Arabic text on this subject and is generally reflective of Islamic efforts to clarify distinctions between categories of madness. He regularly grounded his understanding of mental disorders in humoral pathology and aimed to identify distinct syndromes based on clusters of symptoms that revealed the underlying pathology. Among other conditions linked to brain dysfunction, he discussed phrenitis, lethargy, forgetfulness, epilepsy, apoplexy, and lovesickness. Of all the mental disorders he considered, melancholia and mania were the most emblematic. These conditions were viewed as chronic and non-febrile mental disturbances that expressed two different states; mania generally reflected excited psychotic behavior, while melancholia was associated with a depressed state. Under each of these categories he recognized different sub-categories of the disease. For example, rabies was viewed as a form of mania, while lycanthropy (a condition in which the victim behaves like a rooster and cries like a dog, wanders among tombs in a graveyard at night, and has a yellow complexion, and a dry mouth) was a form of melancholia.

Considering mental illness to be the result of humoral imbalances, Islamic physicians resorted to the same kinds of treatments as they might apply to physical disorders. The careful regulation of diet and regimen was crucial for the *majnun* and various drugs might be prescribed, and bloodletting or cautery could be applied to restore sanity. Even conditions deemed incurable might be palliated through the judicious use of these treatments. Bathing with scented oils, massage, and sexual intercourse were also suggested as beneficial for those suffering from different forms of madness. In medieval Islamic society, some hospitals were developed specifically for the purpose of providing care to the insane. In most cases, however, family members provided for the care of the mentally ill at home, perhaps resorting to hospitals and physicians for medical advice and prescriptions. In this way, despite the efforts of physicians to medicalize the diagnosis and treatment of mental illness, the family and society continued to play the primary role in attending those suffering from mental disorders.

## MENTAL ILLNESS IN MEDIEVAL EUROPE

The scholastic theologian Thomas Aquinas (1225–1274) succinctly summarized what he believed were the three possible causes that might lead people to fall into trances or display unusual mental behaviors:

> First, from a bodily cause, as is clear from those who through some infirmity are out of their minds. Second, through the power of demons, as is seen in those who are possessed. Third, from the divine power. It is in this sense that we speak of ecstasy, when one is elevated to a supernatural level by the divine spirit, with the abstraction from the senses. (Caciola 2003, 33)

Aquinas's thoughts reveal the diverse views of mental illness in medieval society. His writings indicate that he did not view mental disorders as a specifically medical problem, but rather as a social concern that was most appropriately handled by members of the clergy. Indeed, it appears that during the Middle Ages the task of diagnosing and treating mental illness fell mostly into the hands of the family and the local priests, and only rarely were medical professionals called in to offer testimony (e.g., in legal cases) confirming or repudiating diagnoses of mental disorders made by laymen.

Among theologians like Thomas Aquinas, perhaps the primary concern when faced with people manifesting mental disorders was to determine whether it was brought on by divine or demonic possession. Divine madness was viewed positively and was attributed to a divine ecstasy triggered by divine possession or the touch of God; these individuals were often seen as holy fools or even revered for their sanctity and their words were interpreted as revealing God's intentions. By contrast, demonic possession was a sign of the sufferer's weakness and sinfulness and such a person would be distrusted. The difficulty, according to Aquinas and other theologians, was how to determine whether the individual possession was of divine or demonic origin. Both kinds of possession manifested the same external signs, including shrieking and shouting, alienation of the senses, antisocial behavior, entering trancelike or catatonic states, crying, or other displays of grief or despondency. Some suggested that external, bodily signs could be considered to help solve the dilemma, but in general the local community, often with the assistance of the local priest, would make the determination based on a variety of individual factors indicating whether or not they trusted the afflicted.

The treatment of the mentally ill typically remained in the hands of the family and the local community. Families could seek religious cures, and numerous shrines had reputations for offering cures to epileptics and others suffering from mental disorders. In extreme cases, priests might intervene to exorcise demons from the possessed. For example, one man, who displayed signs of mental illness, was brought to a monastery, where the monks tried several methods to exorcise the demon until, "one day [a monk] put the psalter over the head of the possessed man, with him screaming and frothing . . . and after an hour he came to his senses . . . crying out that he had been liberated from the devil" (Caciola 2003, 233). At times, people resorted to harsh methods for treating insane family members, as in the case of a woman in the city of Ferrara, who was said to fill the whole city with terror:

> She gave terrible bites with her teeth to the hands and feet of anyone who was able to catch her. She hurled insults and curses at everyone, mixing in terrible slanders. She threw her body about in almost unspeakable and foul ways. She even tried to burn down her house. . . . [Her family] became impatient and fed up with this, and since they could find no other solution, they tied her up with a strong chain like a dog, and concealed her in a corner of a certain house, so that she could not harm anyone. (Caciola 2003, 46)

By the fourteenth century, hospitals started to segregate the insane from other patients and some hospitals were even established solely for the insane. The mentally ill were often chained up or confined in separate rooms in these hospitals, to isolate them from society, and people could pay to house their mentally ill family members in these institutions. In most cases, however, the mentally ill remained in their own communities and were cared for as holy fools or otherwise incorporated into society as much as possible.

Despite the fact that people in medieval Europe did not typically turn to medical practitioners to treat the mentally ill, learned physicians wrote extensively about how to distinguish and treat different forms of mental disorders. Following Galen, medieval physicians explained mental illness in terms of an imbalance of humors, distinguishing four main categories based on the specific humor that was in excess: frenzy, mania, melancholy, and lethargy. Mental illnesses were, therefore, treated in the same way that other humoral imbalances would be treated—with dietary changes, bloodletting, or drugs—but some physicians advocated other forms of treatment like using sooth-ing words and baths, or trying different means to frighten the patient and shock them into normal behavior, and occasionally trephination (cutting a small hole in the skulls) was prescribed to release heat and other harmful substances accumulating on the brain. Mania, for exam-ple, was thought to be caused by excess yellow bile that dried and heated the brain causing uncontrollable activity, shouting, and violent behavior; it was to be treated with its qualitative opposites, moistening and cooling medicines that would counteract the excess yellow bile.

In the thirteenth and fourteenth centuries, physicians became par-ticularly interested in the disease *amor heroicus* (lovesickness). Those who suffered from this obsessive, unrequited love could be recog-nized by their desiccated and jaundiced appearance, mood swings, characteristic pathetic sighing, loss of appetite, and difficulty sleep-ing; untreated, it could lead to death. During the Middle Ages early discourse on *amor heroicus* tended to localize it in the brain, and mainly emphasized its effects on aristocratic men, who were brought low and even feminized by their excessive desire for the beloved. Later physicians also considered women's susceptibility to this condition, arguing that they were less rational and more desirous of intercourse and, therefore, less able to ward off their amorous desires. Cures were often designed to soothe the body and distract the mind; baths, music, travel, good food, and wine were all recommended, and some phy-sicians even suggested therapeutic intercourse with someone other than the object of obsession.

Another mental illness that received increasing interest in the later Middle Ages was the condition of melancholy. Marsilio Ficino (1433–1499) in his *De vita libri tres* (*Three Books on Life*) offered medical and astrological advice for how to maintain health and prolong life. In par-ticular, he was concerned with the afflictions peculiar to students and scholars, who spend their time in deep contemplation and fail to be sufficiently active. These factors combined to make students especially prone to developing an excess of black bile, which would lead to mel-ancholy. He noted that astrological factors (the influence of Mercury and Saturn) already tend to dry out and cool the brain, and,

> Furthermore, because of the frequent movement involved in thinking, the spirit also is continually broken by such movement. . . . It all comes down to this, that with the mind and heart bent on contemplation, the stomach and the liver fail. Then, especially if you are eating rich or hard foods poorly cooked, the blood becomes cold, thick, and black. Finally, with an excessive swiftness of the limbs, and with neither the remain-ing stuff nor the hard glutinous stuff being separated, dusky vapors are

exhaled. All these make for a melancholy spirit, a sad and fearful soul. . . .
Of all scholars, those devoted to the study of philosophy are most both-
ered by black bile, because their minds get separated from their bodies and from bodily things. They become preoccupied with incorporeal
things, because their work is so much more difficult and the mind
requires an even stronger will. To the extent that they join the mind to
bodiless truth, they are forced to separate it from the body. Body for
these people never returns except as a half-soul and a melancholy one.
(Boer 1980, 7)

In addition to being inactive, even lethargic, Ficino claims that melan-
cholics appear sad due to their quiet, pensive natures and often share
many of the symptoms associated with lovesickness. Overwhelmed
by his deep thoughts and the belief that his uncle Claudius had killed
his father, married his mother, and usurped his throne, Hamlet displays all of the signs of a melancholic. He contemplates death and displays an erratic, pensive nature, with dramatic mood swings, leading
some of the characters to diagnose him, wrongly, as suffering from
lovesickness! Yet, as a melancholic, despite the fact that the ghost of
his father provided a direct imperative to kill Claudius, for most of the
play Hamlet is unable to move himself from thought into *action* and
kill his uncle.

# CHAPTER 10

# The Apothecary and His Pharmacopeia

From the earliest times, people in all societies have recognized the physiological effects of imbibing various local plants, minerals, and other substances. They would have soon recognized those that were toxic, those that caused purgation and those that might have narcotic effects. As people noted these physiological effects, they also began to attribute medicinal virtues to the substances that caused them. Furthermore, some substances without easily recognizable physiological effects were still deemed to have medicinal virtues because of their monetary value, or perceived magical and religious affinities. Increasingly, people began to prepare compound medicines by mixing multiple ingredients in different amounts, tailored to the individual and the disease. In this chapter, we will examine the activities of apothecaries and doctors and the theories that directed their preparation and application of medicinal substances.

## THE PHARMACOPEIA OF ANCIENT MESOPOTAMIA

The *Epic of Gilgamesh* relates how the hero, Gilgamesh, went on a quest to find a cure for his friend, Enkidu, who was suffering from a deadly illness. He learned about a secret healing plant that was supposed to ward off decay and rejuvenate all who consumed it, and he swam to the bottom of deep waters to recover it. After returning to shore,

Gilgamesh fell asleep and a snake ate the healing plant and gained the power to rejuvenate itself by sloughing off its old skin. Upon awakening, Gilgamesh wept, recognizing that he had lost this most precious plant that offered the power to cure the ills of mankind.

Gilgamesh's quest reveals the Mesopotamian recognition of the healing attributes of plants, whose powers were unknown to most men. The *asu*, however, was known for his use of drugs to cure disease; his pharmacopeia included a range of plants (seeds, roots, leaves, bark, resin, and flowers), parts of animals (including dung), and some minerals. Many of these substances produced observable effects (acting as emetics, purgatives, or expectorants), suggesting to the *asu* that they were working, even if modern physicians are doubtful of their therapeutic efficacy. Obtaining the exact ingredients was believed to be very important for the success of the remedy. One *asu* makes this clear in a letter to his lord, requesting new herbs:

> The daughter of Mustalu who was coughing but not spitting out has started to expectorate after I gave her [appropriate] potions; but . . . now she is constipated. I gave her a potion for constipation to drink, and she is taking it, (but) there is no *sarmadu* herb and drawn wine available. Let my lord send (some) so that I can have her drink, lest she develop "Hand of Curse." The princess who had repeated attacks of fever has now calmed thanks to the dressing and potion. As to the herbs of which I spoke to my lord, let my lord not forget about them. (Biggs 2005, 12)

These medicinal substances would be prepared in various ways depending on the illness (e.g., being crushed, cooked, or dried) and then put into a drink (water, milk, beer, or wine) to create a healing potion or mixed with other substances (e.g., honey, ash, or flour) to create a poultice for external application on wounds or burns.

The Mesopotamian *asu* also provided medicines for cosmetic reasons, such as combating hair loss or turning gray hair black. Cures listed under headings such as, "If a man's head in his youth is full of grey hairs, to darken the grey hair . . ." listed a range of ingredients such as the gall of a black ox or the fat of a black raven, suggesting that the color of the substance used would be transferred to the hair. In one remedy, the *asu* is told to crush those or similar substances in oil of the cypress from a cemetery and then explains, "the charm seven times thou shalt recite . . . , [under] the stars thou shalt set it, (on) his head press it, bind on for seven days and he shall recover" (Thompson 1924, 12). These remedies suggest the importance of magical affinities in the selection of ingredients and in the application cures. The need to recite a charm along with the specifications for the conditions in which the compound should be applied should remind us that magic and medicine were closely united in Mesopotamian society.

## THE EGYPTIAN PHARMACOPEIA

Providing medicinal substances was the most common form of treatment recommended in the Egyptian medical papyri. Indeed, Egyptian doctors were renowned in neighboring countries for their pharmaceutical expertise. The *Odyssey*, for example, indicates the high esteem of Egyptian pharmaceutical lore among the Greeks in one passage where an Egyptian woman provides a drug to ease pain: "potent gifts from Polydamna the wife of Thon, a woman of Egypt, land where the teeming soil bears the richest yield of herbs in all the world: many health itself when mixed in the wine, and many deadly poison. Every man is a healer there, more skilled than any other men on earth—Egyptians born of the healing god himself" (Fagles 1996, 131).

The Egyptian *swnw* used a variety of plant, animal, and mineral substances in his efforts to prepare drugs. In many cases, we are unable to identify exactly what substance the Egyptian doctors meant, whether because we cannot link a specific plant to the name, or because the substance is simply too fantastical (e.g., "excrement-of-the-gods"). Many of the prescriptions are simple, with only one drug taken, but the majority are compound medicines with anywhere from half a dozen to a dozen drugs, and in one case, as many as thirty-seven different substances! The ingredients are typically mixed with different delivery vehicles including water, milk, beer, and wine to make healing potions. Even here, however, several distinctions are made so that the *swnw* might use, for example, warm beer, flat beer, sweet beer, fresh milk, spoiled milk, warm milk, milk-of-a-woman-who-has-borne-a-son, well water, spring water, salt water, or water-in-which-the-phallus-has-been-washed. Medicines were often given orally as pills, gargles, or potions, or applied externally as ointments or poultices. They could also be provided by fumigation, directing the steam or smoke from the cooking or burning medicine into the affected area. Finally, many drugs were administered rectally or vaginally as an enema or suppository.

Prescriptions are often accompanied with an explanation for their magical efficacy, or with an explanation justifying their use in terms of disease theory. In many cases, medicines were applied to purge the pathological *wekhedu* (a morbid or disease-causing principle believed to originate in the anus) from the body. The Ebers papyrus offers a remedy, using an unknown herb (*senutet*):

> Beginning of remedies to cause mucus to go down from the pelvis. A
> herb—*senutet* is its name—growing on its belly like the *kadet*-plant. It
> produces a flower like the lotus. If one finds its leaves [looking] like
> white wood, then one should fetch it and rub it on the pelvis. Then it
> (the mucus) will go down immediately. Its fruit is given on bread to
> [those with] *wekhedu* to cause (it) to go down from the pelvis. (Nunn
> 1996, 128–139)

In fact, the ancient Egyptians were continually worried about the possibility of decay brought on by *wekhedu*, especially in the anus, and
many prescriptions (indeed, one entire medical papyrus) are devoted
specifically to remedies for refreshing or cooling the anus and "to drive
out excrement." Indeed, one Greek historian, Herodotus, observed that
Egyptians regularly sought to use emetics and laxatives, noting that
"for three days in succession in each month they physic themselves,
hunting health with emetics and purges, because they think that from
the food that nourishes mankind come all their diseases" (Grene 1987,
163). Various parts of the castor oil tree were considered especially useful as laxatives, as one remedy makes clear: "When a person who suffers from constipation chews a little of its [the castor oil tree's] berry
along with beer, then the disease will be driven out of the sick one's
body." In addition to castor oil, Egyptians used a variety of substances
as laxatives including dates, figs, coriander, cumin, wormwood, or mal-
achite combined with other ingredients (Bryan 1974, 16).

Egyptian pharmacology was also important for cosmetic and domestic applications. Remedies were provided to combat hair loss or gray
hair, to drive away wrinkles, remove moles or even to cure sweaty feet.
The Egyptians were also masters of making eye paints, which they
offered to gods (painting the eyes of the statues of gods with them)
or as cosmetics. Eye paints were prescribed by the *swnw* not only for
aesthetic purposes, but also as medicines to treat a variety of eye diseases. Indeed, the Ebers papyrus has a section devoted to remedies for
*wekhedu* collecting with blood in the eyes, which describes a number
of eye paints that can be applied around the eyes or directly on the
eyes. Finally, the *swnw*'s pharmacopeia also had other uses around the
household to give clothes a pleasant fragrance or to drive away ver-
min. One text suggests this remedy to keep mice away from clothes:
use cat's fat and smear it on everything possible!

## GREEK AND ROMAN PHARMACOLOGY

The Hippocratic authors left no single pharmacological book or herbal
manual describing various drugs, their preparation, and application.

Indeed, the favored therapy in Hippocratic medicine was the regulation of diet and regimen, and the use of drugs takes on a secondary role in therapeutics. When Hippocratic texts prescribe drugs, they are most often simple remedies (those composed of a single ingredient), which are most often prescribed for their effects as purgatives or emetics. For example, black hellebore is prescribed as a purgative while mixtures of wine and honey are offered to ease coughs and act as expectorants.

A number of specialized herbals were written in the Roman period. One of the earliest of these, the *Compositiones* (*Prescriptions*) by Scribonius Largus (ca. 1–50 C.E.) describes 271 recipes that mix plant, mineral, and animal ingredients found in regions around the Mediterranean or imported from further east. The text is divided into three parts with the first part giving remedies for diseases organized from head-to-toe, followed by a section with antidotes against poisons, bites, and stings, and a final section on plasters and wound dressings. Plant products (including carrots, aloe, fenugreek and ginger) are most common, but he also prescribes the use of animals and minerals—his remedy for a constant headache is to touch an electric ray or torpedo fish, since the constant shocks would help suppress the pain.

One of Scribonius's contemporaries, Pliny the Elder (23–79 C.E.), also wrote about the medicinal uses of plants, animals, and minerals in his *Natural History*. Pliny drew his information largely from other Greek and Latin sources on pharmacology and he covers a much wider range of ingredients than Scribonius. His large text describes the therapeutic properties of each ingredient, some of which seem to suggest magical powers. For example, he notes the remedies that can be derived from rosemary:

> A local application of the fresh root heals wounds . . . and hemorrhoids. The juice both of the shrub and of the root cures jaundice and such conditions as call for cleansing. . . . The seed is given in drink for chronic complaints of the chest and with wine and pepper for uterine trouble . . . an application also clears away freckles. . . . The herb itself is applied with vinegar to scrofulous sores, and with honey is good for a cough. (Jones 1956, 73)

And, from the elephant,

> The blood of an elephant, particularly that of the male, checks all the fluxes that are called *rheumatismi*. Ivory shavings with Attic honey are said to remove dark spots on the face, and ivory dust whitlows. By the touch of the trunk headache is relieved, more successfully if the animal also sneezes. The right side of the trunk used as an amulet with the red

earth of Lemnos is aphrodisiac. The blood too is good for consumption, and the liver for epilepsy. (Jones 1963, 63)

Pliny also describes various medical conditions and their treatments. These conditions range from poisoning, to ulcers and fistulas, eye diseases, fevers, coughs, and warts. Pliny's work was valued for its breadth of coverage, but it is highly disorganized and later generations of physicians complained about his willingness to include rumors and hearsay in his accounts.

Perhaps the most successful pharmacological text from Greco-Roman antiquity was the *De Materia Medica* by Dioscorides of Anazarbus (ca. 40–90 c.e.). This herbal, divided into five books, describes the medicinal

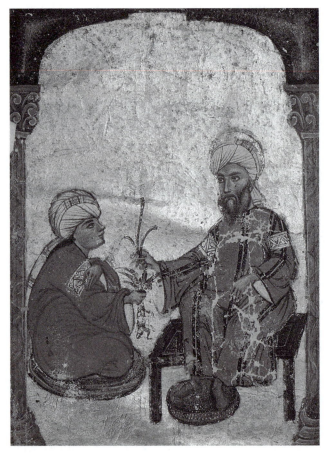

This scene from an Arabic translation of Dioscorides's *Materia Medica* from 1228 depicts Dioscorides teaching herb lore to a student. (Werner Forman Archive/StockphotoPro)

properties of over a thousand substances, including around seven hundred plants, as well as minerals and animal products. He also explains the proper means of harvesting and storing plants for medicinal use. Throughout, Dioscorides claims that he had actively sought out and tested the recipes he describes:

> [I], . . . having an unceasing desire to acquire knowledge of this matter, and having travelled much (for you know that I led a soldier's life), have by your advice gathered together all that I have commented hereupon . . . But I beg that you, and all who may peruse these commentaries, will not pay attention so much to the force of our words, as to the industry and experience that I have brought to bear in the matter. For with very accurate diligence, knowing most herbs with mine own eyes, others by historical relations agreeable to all, and by questioning, diligently enquiring of the inhabitants of each sort, we will endeavor . . . to describe the kinds and forces of every one of them. (Gunther 1959, 2)

Still, many of his remedies may seem rather strange or unappetizing: "House mice, being cut asunder, are applied profitably to those who are stung by scorpions . . . [and] being eaten roasted they do dry the spittle in the mouths of children" (Gunther 1959, 308). His herbal became the main source for pharmaceutical knowledge for the next fifteen centuries, and it was translated from the original Greek into many languages including Latin, Arabic, and English, and many later editions included numerous colorful illustrations of the plants described.

Most of the medicines described in the Greek and Roman herbals were fairly simple, typically composed of a single substance, but at most consisting of only a few ingredients. The complexity of drug preparation increased as the selection of ingredients rose, especially in the larger cities in the later Roman Empire. The most visible example of this was the development of the compound medicines that could serve as antidotes for snakebite and other poisons. Pliny relates the story of king Mithridates VI of Pontus (120–63 B.C.E.), who developed a poison antidote composed of forty-one ingredients, which was later named "Mithridatium." In the first century C.E., Nero's personal physician, Andromachus, revised the formula to include sixty-four ingredients, adding viper flesh and increasing the proportion of opiates; he dedicated his recipe for "theriac" (also known as "treacle" in English) to Nero. In the next century, Galen further revised the recipe for theriac, which he prescribed for the emperor Marcus Aurelius, to include seventy-seven ingredients listed in his *De theriaca ad Pisonem*. In later centuries, theriac was used not only as an antidote for poisons, but also as a powerful panacea, prescribed for a wide range of conditions until the nineteenth century.

## PHARMACY IN AYURVEDIC MEDICINE

Pharmaceutical remedies provide an important cornerstone of Indian medicine. The Ayurvedic texts emphasize the importance of the *pañca-karman* ("five procedures") therapy for restoring the appropriate levels of the *doshas* in the body. The five procedures are the administration of emetics (*vanuna*), purgatives (*virecana*), enemas (*basti*), errhines (*nasya*, to promote sneezing), and bloodletting (*raktamokshana*). In theory, emetics are used to evacuate excess *doshas* orally, especially for ailments caused by *kapha* (phlegm); purgatives are used to eliminate *doshas* and *malas* (sweat, urine, and feces) from the lower parts of the body and especially in ailments caused by *pitta* (bile); rectal and vaginal enemas are used in cases of fevers, diarrhea, constipation, and flatulence; and errhines are used for ailments of the head, neck, ears, nose, and throat. These therapeutic actions are only supposed to be undertaken after the patient has undergone oleation (the application of medicated oils externally and internally) and sudation (sweating). The preliminary measures are taken to eliminate impurities from the body that might block the *srotas* (channels) in the body and hence cause illness and disrupt the healing action of the drugs.

The *Susruta* alone mentions over seven hundred medicinal herbs, not to mention mineral and animal products, and later texts add many others. The medicinal properties of these substances were classified according to the six basic *rasa* (tastes): sweet, sour, salty, pungent, bitter, and astringent.

> Sweet taste increases all *dhatus, ojas*, semen and breast-milk; is beneficial for eyes, hair and complexion . . . if it is used regularly alone and in excess, it produces the following diseases—cough, dyspnoea, [flatulence], vomiting, sweetness in mouth, loss of voice. . . . Sour is digestive for food as well as *dosha, ama* or inflammation; stimulates digestive fire, pacifies *vatta*, is carminative, produces burning in bowels, is externally cold, moistening and mostly relishing; in spite of having such properties, if it is used regularly alone and in excess, it produces tingling of teeth, blinking of eyes . . . causes suppuration in wounds, injuries, burns, bites, fractures and dislocations. . . . Astringent taste is anti-diarrheal, healing, stiffening, cleansing, scraping, absorbent and pressing and dries up moisture; in spite of having such properties, if used for a long time alone and in excess, it produces cardiac pain, dryness of mouth, flatulence, loss of speech, [stiff neck], quivering in body parts, tingling sensation, contraction, convulsion. (Sharma 1999, 389–391)

However, the taste of each substance was often interpreted as a combination of two or more of the basic flavors, requiring careful efforts to produce compound drugs with the appropriate balance of flavors. Substances were further classified as "hot" or "cold" depending upon the feeling that they produced in the body.

There are several methods for preparing drugs in Ayurvedic medicine. Medical texts discuss the knowledge necessary for growing and properly harvesting medicinal plants to maximize their efficacy. Once collected, plants would be prepared as drugs in a variety of forms (as pastes, juices, cold infusions, hot infusions, or decoctions), and the correct form to prescribe needed to be determined "with due regard to the strength of the patient and seriousness of the disease [since] all these preparations are not equally useful in all cases" (Sharma and Dash 1976, 85). In addition to producing these extractions, infusions, and decoctions, plants were also ground into powders or mixed with oils or other liquids to produce pastes or plasters, or prepared as pills or suppositories. Given the religious restrictions enforced by Brahmans in Hindu society, it is perhaps surprising that the *vaidya* did not restrict his prescriptions in accordance with taboos against the use of animal products in drugs, and even prescribed alcoholic drinks.

## Siddha Medicine and Alchemical Remedies

A system of medicine developed in the Tamil-speaking regions in south India that was different in some respects from Ayurvedic medicine. Known as Siddha medicine, this system was taught by the legendary Siddhas, "Perfect Ones," who were portrayed as combining the practices of yoga and alchemy. It is strongly influenced by tantric thought and distinguishes itself from Ayurveda by its emphasis on the examination of the pulse and by the greater use of metal-based and alchemical remedies. The classical Sanskrit texts devoted to *rasayana* ("the way of the *rasas*," or alchemy) date from about the tenth century C.E. and treat the production of healing or rejuvenating elixirs, as well the practices of transmutational alchemy. These texts view mercury as the essence (*rasa*) of all other substances and, therefore, it was the prime alchemical reagent studied and an important medicinal substance. The Siddha medical and alchemical texts also hold the substance called *muppa*, which seems to have been similar to the "philosopher's stone" pursued by Western alchemists, in particular reverence since it was believed capable of bringing about both physical and spiritual transformations. The Siddha pharmacopoeia, therefore, makes greater use of mineral and metallic ingredients than Ayurvedic medicine, but it also attaches importance to the use of medicinal plants.

## THE TRADITIONAL CHINESE PHARMACOPEIA

### Early Materia Medica

Works on materia medica spread among the people of China even prior to the Han dynasty (206 B.C.E.–220 C.E.), but most have been lost. Like the *Wu-shih-erh ping fang* (*Fifty-Two Prescriptions against Fifty-Two Ailments*), unearthed in the Mawangdui tombs from ca. 168 B.C.E., these texts likely contained lists of various pharmaceutical products that could be applied for different conditions. Although these texts list individual remedies and sometimes offer a theoretical justification for their use, they do not attempt a systematic consideration of pharmacy.

The earliest extant treatise to provide a theoretical classification of the ingredients in the materia medica was the *Shen Nong Ben Cao Jing* (*Shen Nong's Classic of Materia Medica*), produced sometime in the first century C.E. It lists 365 drugs of plant (252), animal (67) and mineral (46) origin, which were classified into three grades or potencies: superior, average and inferior. Superior drugs (120 kinds, including ginseng), were deemed non-toxic and were used as tonics for long-term treatment to produce an invigorating effect. By contrast, the average drugs (120 kinds, including Chinese angelica) were toxic in some cases and could be used as tonics to help resist disease or expel unhealthy pathogens from the body. Finally, the inferior drugs (125 kinds, including croton), many of which were recognized as toxic, were prescribed in drastic cases to help expel harmful materials from the body and were not meant to be taken for prolonged periods. The properties of each drug were carefully described as in the case of ginseng, which was said to have, "the quality of tonifying the five viscera (*zang*), relieving mental stress . . . ending palpitation, removing pathogenic Cold and Heat, improving acuity of sight, enlightening and benefitting the brain, [assisting] longevity and pleasing and relaxing the mood when taken over a long period" (Zhenguo, Ping, and Peiping 1999, 64). In addition to classifying the drugs and describing their therapeutic properties, the text also addresses problems of harvesting, processing and storing the various ingredients and how they can be combined in compound medicines, including explanations for adding ingredients that could diminish the toxic side effects of others. The *Shen Nong Ben Cao Jing* was recognized for its utility and quickly became the primary pharmaceutical text in China.

### Alchemy and Pharmaceutical Chemistry

The spread of Taoism had an important influence on the development of alchemical medicine in ancient China. Taoist doctrines encouraged a return to a simpler way of life and the pursuit of harmony with nature, and for some this pursuit led to a search for immortality. Taoist thought had greatly influenced the development of herbal medicine, but it also encouraged the study of alchemy. The Taoist adept, Ge Hong (ca. 281–341 C.E.), known also by his pseudonym, Baopuzi, was perhaps the most eminent alchemist to turn his interest toward medical applications in his pursuit of drugs to prolong life. He worked mostly with cinnabar (the principle ore of mercury) and other mineral and metallic substances (sulphur, realgar, saltpeter, alum, mica, iron, tin, and gold) in alchemical experiments, but he also studied medicinal plants. He summarized his alchemical experiments in the *Bao Pu Zi Nei Pian* (*Bao Pu Zi's Inner Treatise*), which included many alchemical drugs for the purpose of producing longevity, like this one:

> The Lesser Divine elixir: Take three pounds of real cinnabar, six pounds of white honey, stir together, expose to the sun, and cook until it can be shaped into pills. Every morning take ten of these pills about the size of a hempseed. In less than a year, whitened hair will become black, lost teeth will regrow, and the skin of your whole body be moist and rejuvenated. Those who take it will not age, and old men will regain their youths, enjoy Fullness of Life, and become immortal. (Ware 1966, 95, 188)

Tao Hongjing (452–536 C.E.), another Taoist physician, also aimed to combine the alchemical tradition with medical pharmacy. In addition to writing several works on alchemy, Tao Hongjing wrote a commentary on the *Shen Nong Ben Cao Jing* in an effort to correct the mistakes he found in it. His *Ben Cao Jing Ji Zhu* (*Collective Notes to the Classic of Materia Medica*), quoted the original *Shen Nong Ben Cao Jing* in red ink with a supplementary commentary in black ink printed alongside in order to facilitate interpretation and help highlight corrections. He also added 365 drugs to those already described in the *Shen Nong Ben Cao Jing* (730 altogether) and revised the classification system so that they were first divided into categories based on their origin (jade and stone, plant, insect and animal, fruit, vegetable, cereal, and others) before further organizing them according to their medicinal grades (superior, average, and inferior). Tao Hongjing's classification system became the standard method for organizing drugs in Chinese medicine for more than 1,000 years.

## Standardizing Materia Medica and Regulating the Drug Market

Shortly after the national unification under the Tang dynasty (618–907 C.E.), the imperial government perceived the need for an official pharmacopeia. Emperor Gaozong asked the physician Su Jing to evaluate previous pharmaceutical manuals and produce a revised and corrected materia medica. Starting in 657, Su Jing led a group of over twenty scholars, and augmented Tao Hongjing's *Ben Cao Jing Ji Zhu* with more than one hundred new drugs. Completed in 659, the *Xin Xiu Ben Cao* (*Newly-Compiled Materia Medica*), later known as the *Tang Ben Cao* (*Materia Medica of the Tang*), was the first government sponsored pharmacopeia in the world and became the standard pharmaceutical reference manual in China for the next 300 years. The original version included several volumes of illustrations, which are unfortunately now lost. Among other things, this book contains the first recorded description of a silver electuary (made of tin, silver foil, and mercury) for dental fillings.

The imperial court of the Song dynasty (960–1279 C.E.) was also extremely concerned with the regulation of pharmacological texts, especially given the rapid proliferation of these texts allowed by the introduction of woodblock printing. In response, the court established the Bureau for the Re-Editing of Medical Books to oversee the revision and printing of classical medical textbooks. The Bureau was also charged toward the end of the tenth century C.E. with the production of the *Taiping Sheng Hui Fang* (*Peaceful Holy Benevolent Formulas*), a formulary listing 16,834 prescriptions for compound medicines that drew together and standardized material from previous texts on pharmacology. The Song government also implemented a large-scale investigation of drugs from around the country, which resulted in the publication of the *Ben Cao Tu Jing* (*Illustrated Classic of Materia Medica*) in 1061, the first extant illustrated pharmacopeia from China. The book contained folk remedies and proven herbal drugs with 933 illustrations to assist in their proper identification.

The Song imperial court also organized the first official institute to oversee the manufacture and sale of drugs in 1076 and by 1103 six new dispensaries had been established in different parts of China. These drug-processing workshops were responsible for collecting, testing, manufacturing, and selling drugs, and for dispensing medicines to the poor in times of medical emergency. The Institute also printed its own formulary that included 788 prescriptions (far more manageable than the list in the *Taiping Sheng Hui Fang*) in the *He Ji Ju Fang* (*Prescriptions Collected by the Pharmaceutical Institute*).

## PHARMACY IN THE ISLAMIC WORLD

Islamic pharmacy relied heavily on the Greek tradition, especially on the works of Dioscorides and Galen's treatise *On the Powers of Simple Drugs*. These works were increasingly available in Arabic translation from the tenth century onward. However, the Greek materia medica were limited in that the plants they described were frequently unknown in many parts of the Middle East, although local related species could sometimes be identified. At the same time the wide geographic range of the Islamic world (from Spain, across North Africa, and into the Middle East) and the extended trade routes that reached as far as India and China meant that Islamic authors came into contact with many new drugs that had not been described by their Greek forebears. So, while the Greek texts offered a theoretical framework within which to consider drug therapy, Islamic authors wrote numerous original pharmacological treatises.

One of the most common genres of pharmacological literature were the synonymic lists of drugs, providing equivalent names in different languages such as Greek, Latin, Syriac, Persian, Hindi, Berber, and Spanish, to aid in the proper identification of plants. For example, Maimonides (d. 1204), one of the most famous Jewish scholars writing in Arabic, composed a list containing 408 well-known drugs with their synonyms, like this entry on *ratina* ("resin"):

> This is the resin which the people of the Maghrib [Berbers] call *rajina* and the people of Egypt *qulfuniya*. It is also called *zaft al-ghadhawa*. It is the resin of the male pine or of the dry terebinth. On the contrary, the resin called κολοφωυια in ancient Greek is the resin of the small pine which is not *al-qulfuniya*. (Levey 1966, 8)

In addition to clarifying the local names for plants described in the Greek texts, these lists might offer suggestions for possible substitutes.

Islamic authors also wrote original treatises on materia medica. These typically presented drugs in alphabetical order for ease of reference and generally include a description of the plant, a discussion of its preparation and therapeutic use, and a summary of the opinions about the drug from various authorities. Probably the best-known manual of this kind is Ibn al-Baytar's (d. 1248) *Comprehensive Book on Simple Drugs and Foodstuffs*, which lists over 1,400 drugs. Al-Baytar reports his own observations about the medicinal value of many of these drugs and also draws upon over 260 written sources, augmenting the Greek and Roman pharmacopeia with many new items discovered through

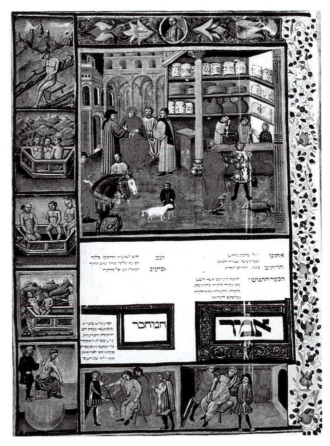

This is a page from a Hebrew manuscript copy of Avicenna's *Canon* from about 1440. The central scene depicts a university-trained physician (in his red academic gown) meeting patients during his office hours. In the foreground another physician meets a messenger carrying a basket used to transport a urine sample; physicians claimed to be able to diagnose a patient's condition from their urine, without having to see him or her in person. Both physicians are conveniently located next to an apothecary's shop (with its shelves lined with containers for medicinal herbs) where patients could fill their prescriptions. During the Middle Ages, some physicians had arrangements with local apothecaries to share profits from drug sales. Smaller images around the edge depict other forms of therapeutics, including balneology (baths), cupping, bloodletting, and surgery (perhaps to lance a boil). (National Library of Medicine)

practice and in exchanges with India and China, including camphor, musk, senna, and cotton (which was prescribed for use in wound dressings).

Several Arabic pharmacological treatises focused exclusively on poisons. These texts consider the dangers of bites by various insects, snakes and mad dogs, as well as the stings of scorpions, and the poisonous properties of various minerals and plants. A typical example was the *Kitab al-sumum* (*Book on Poisons*) by Ibn Wahshiyah (fl. before 912), which describes a number of poisons and venoms. For example, he observes that some people use a particular species of blister fly deceitfully as a poison, mixing it with food or drink. Anyone, he says, who imbibes the fly in this way will experience burning in his throat, a violent stomachache, abdominal swelling and sometimes the suppression of urination and bowel movements, concluding that "this animal is fatal in one day and no later." He suggests a number of antidotes, including the following: "To save the poison victim quickly, the best remedy is to suck milk from the breast of a woman many times. He sucks, stops, sucks, and stops continuously until his belly symptoms disappear. If he is anointed with pure violet oil, it is useful for him" (Levey 1966, 9–10).

Islamic authors also wrote formularies, which provided recipes for mixing compound medicines. Such texts were usually organized according to the kind of compound produced (pill, syrup, powder, gargle, emetic, suppository, poultice, etc.) and described the conditions for which it could be used. Formularies could be appended to other medical texts or circulate independently, like al-Kindi's (d. after 870) *Aqrabadhin* (*Prescriptions*), and they appear to have been produced frequently for use in hospital dispensaries, such as the formulary by the Jewish apothecary, Ibn Abi al-Bayan (d. ca. 1240), who practiced in the famous Nasir hospital in Cairo, Egypt.

## MEDIEVAL EUROPEAN PHARMACOLOGY

In medieval Europe, the task of preparing and selling drugs was typically undertaken by apothecaries. These tradesmen were often involved in the spice trade and thus able to import exotic substances from all over Europe, the Mediterranean, and the Near East. Although they held a lower status and did not have the theoretical training of the university physicians, apothecaries would also often dispense medical advice and thus served as another class of medical practitioner. The competition among the different kinds of medical practitioners did not always create tensions and in some places apothecaries and physicians entered into mutually beneficial agreements whereby the physician would meet patients in the apothecary's shop and then write prescriptions that could be filled on the premises and for which the physician might receive a percentage. Increasingly, physicians, especially those in university towns, sought to establish their authority to regulate the preparation and sale of drugs. Several physicians reported on the dangers of different medicines, especially laxatives and opiates, and questioned whether apothecaries should be allowed to prepare such drugs without supervision, let alone sell them without a physician's prescription. For example, a physician in Montpellier, Bernard of Gordon (active in the late thirteenth and early fourteenth centuries), recalled a case in which he was called to treat an apothecary who had accidentally suffered an overdose of theriac due to his own negligence:

> It happened that a certain apothecary had sold a toxic substance and some remained behind the nail of his thumb. When he began to pick his nose with his thumb, his color began to change and he fainted repeatedly. When he took three drams [of the antidote, theriac], his condition became more serious. I was called around midnight and I saw that the amount of theriac had been too high. I made him vomit and after he had purged his stomach sufficiently, I gave him one dram of theriac and he was cured. (Demaitre 1980, 76)

Bernard's point here is that apothecaries are not careful in their drug preparation and they do not understand the theory that dictates appropriate dosage for different remedies. Despite the learned physicians' fears, however, apothecaries regularly prepared and sold drugs and offered medical advice throughout Europe.

One reason that university physicians sought to regulate the activities of apothecaries was that they increasingly emphasized the theoretical and technical difficulties of drug preparation in their new pharmacological literature. In particular, physicians aimed to incorporate Galenic theories about simple medicines that categorized them by their primary qualities (hot, cold, wet, or dry), which served as a rational explanation for their actions on a patient's humoral imbalance. In its simplest sense, a patient would be given a medicine qualitatively opposed to the disease, for example, a cold medicine to counteract the effects of a hot disease. However, the theory as it developed was far more complicated. Following Galen and the pharmaceutical writings of Arabic authors like al-Kindi, university physicians argued that medicinal simples (single substances) could be graded in four "degrees" according to the strength of their primary quality. Arnald of Villanova (ca. 1238–ca. 1310), working at the medical school of

Montpellier, elaborated upon this theory and its application in making compound medicines.

> There are many reasons for the compounding of medicines; namely, strength of the disease, contrariety of diseases, contrary disposition of members [parts of the body], . . . [and] violence of the medicine. For certain violent diseases such as leprosy, apoplexy and epilepsy can rarely if at all be cured by simple medicines. Compounds must therefore be used, so that their force may more easily bring about the cure of a violent disease. A compound medicine is also necessary in the case of contrary diseases present in one and the same body, such as a fever [hot disease] and leucophlegmancy [cold disease], where we must employ a medicine compounded from both hot and cold, so that it can act against the opposite diseases. . . . A compound medicine must also be made up in the case of contrary qualities present within the bodily members, as when the stomach is chilled but the liver is heated. Finally, violent medicines, such as scammony, hellebore, and the like, cannot be given simply, but must have others admixed with them to diminish their violence. (McVaugh 1975, 14)

Taking these factors into account, Arnald developed theories for how to mix substances composed of different degrees and different qualities to produce a compound medicine appropriate for the nature of the disease(s) afflicting an individual patient. In theory, this meant that the physician needed to recognize the degree of the patient's complexional imbalance (e.g., a disease might be caused by excess phlegm, cold and wet, in different degrees, depending on its strength) and then mix suitable simples to achieve the appropriate degree to counteract the disease (e.g., a drug hot in the first degree and dry in the second degree). The theory sparked extensive debate and justified physicians' efforts to regulate apothecaries, but in practice it was too complicated and even Arnald's prescriptions suggest that he did not always follow it. In practice, physicians and apothecaries were more likely to tailor prescriptions for compound medicines according to the wealth of the patient (e.g., suggesting less expensive ingredients for poor patients), or the availability of substances, than follow the complex mathematical theory. Nonetheless, this is an early effort aimed at applying mathematical theory in mixing compound drugs.

# CHAPTER 11

# War and Health

Prehistoric humans developed a number of weapons, including fire, spears, and stone clubs, for use as protection against animals and other human tribes. Over time, other weapons were developed that could be used at greater ranges (such as the sling and the bow and arrow) and as humans learned how to work metals they replaced traditional stone tools with bronze weapons that could be easily sharpened, including swords, axes, and bronze tips for spears, javelins, and arrows. Early cave paintings from the Paleolithic period (35,000–12,000 B.C.E.) indicate that humans had begun to employ strategies and tactics that would best use their weapons in combat, creating the first organized warfare. As humans organized into cities and began to deploy larger armies, they began to adopt more systematized policies for composing and deploying their forces, training and arming different groups that might serve as specialized foot soldiers, cavalrymen, archers, or other positions. Each unit would be recognizable based upon its specialized armor and weaponry.

Being wounded in combat was, in many ways, the least of the dangers faced by soldiers in any premodern army. The difficulties of transporting the food necessary to maintain a fighting force in the field meant that soldiers were often left to fend for themselves, scavenging what food they could find from the lands through which they moved, and hunger was ever present. Of even more concern, the sanitary conditions of military life meant that armies were often troubled by a wide range of different diseases, so that a soldier's chance of dying from illness was at least as great as dying from a wound in battle. Civilians faced similar health dangers as invading armies moved through their lands, stealing and destroying crops, raiding and burning villages, and besieging cities.

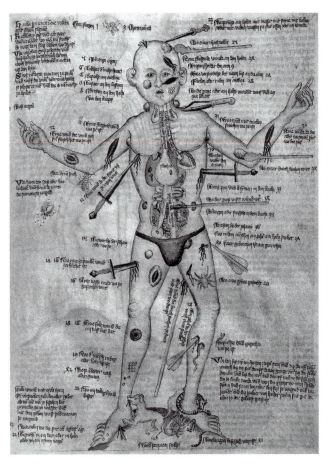

The "wound man" illustration, like this one from around 1420–1430, was common in medieval European surgical manuals. Wound man images depict the numerous wounds a human body could suffer, including sword and knife cuts, crushing blows from clubs, arrow wounds, bites from insects and animals, and various rashes or burns. Some wound man illustrations, like this one, also provided a schematic view of internal organs. (Wellcome Library, London)

## WEAPONS AND WOUNDS

What type of wound was a soldier likely to encounter in battle? The most common weapons used were arrows, sling bullets, swords, axes, maces, spears, and javelins. These weapons produced different kinds of wounds and treatment varied considerably according to the type of injury. Slashing weapons, especially very sharp swords or heavy axes, could produce traumatic amputations (of limbs or heads), but more often they produced flesh wounds, which many surgical authors considered the least dangerous of wounds, so long as they did not contact the bone or cut through nerves and tendons. Piercing wounds from thrusting weapons like swords, arrows, javelins, and spears were usually considered more deadly. For this reason, Roman soldiers were often trained to use their swords as thrusting rather than slashing weapons; as one Roman author noted: "a cut, with whatever violence it may come, does not often kill . . . but, on the other hand, a stab, thrust in two inches deep, is fatal" (Salazar 2000, 12). Weapons like clubs, maces, and war hammers were designed for delivering heavy blows that could crush armor and fracture bones.

The recent excavation of a mass grave near the Towton battlefield in England has allowed archaeologists to examine the variety of wounds soldiers typically experienced in battle (Boylston 2000, 357–380). The Battle of Towton took place during the War of the Roses between King Henry VI of the house of Lancaster and Edward Earl of March of the house of York on March 29, 1461, with over 100,000 combatants and approximately 28,000 deaths. Examination of skeletal remains reveals that many individuals sustained multiple injuries from a variety of projectiles and hand weapons. Blows appear to have been clustered around the head and face, with fewer injuries to the limbs and torso. These findings suggest that the limbs and torso were not targeted as often, that the individuals were wearing armor in those places, or that wounds in those regions were slashing or piercing flesh wounds that did not penetrate to leave marks on the bones. Many of the wounds are quite brutal, with one skeleton revealing that the soldier's jaw had been sliced from his face by a sword that cut through the roots of a molar and almost certainly severed his tongue. Other remains reveal previous injuries that had healed, showing that not all battle wounds were fatal. Interestingly, it appears that some remains show damage to the teeth that would likely have resulted from archers using their teeth to string their bows.

Surgical manuals reveal the kinds of operations battlefield surgeons would have needed to perform in order to attend to this array of wounds. With most wounds, the control of hemorrhage would have been the surgeon's most immediate concern. The application of pressure to the wound was the first recourse, but sometimes the surgeon would need to resort to more extreme measures. The Roman author Celsus (ca. 25 B.C.E.–ca. 50 C.E.), describes two other methods that could be used to stop hemorrhaging:

> But if even these [other procedures] are powerless against the profuse bleeding, the blood-vessels which are pouring out blood are to be seized, and round the wounded spot they are to be tied in two places and cut across between so that the two ends coalesce each on itself and yet have their orifices closed. When circumstances do not even admit of this, the blood-vessels can be burnt with a red-hot iron. (Spencer 1953, 81)

This account by Celsus is one of the earliest of the application of a vascular ligature and it was not an easy procedure to perform, especially on a battlefield. Once the initial bleeding was under control, wounds would be bandaged or closed with sutures.

Closing abdominal gashes required extra attention as attested by the numerous accounts of the operation. Galen (129–ca. 216 C.E.) graphically explains the procedure: "first one needs to put away the prolapsed intestines into their proper place," which "needs a dexterous assistant," then "grasping the entire wound with his hands from the outside, he needs to push it inwards and press it together and present it to the one who is suturing little by little, and then also compress moderately that which has been sutured, until it has been sutured accurately" (Salazar 2000, 51). Sometimes the intestines themselves were sliced and needed to be sutured, as in the case described by the medieval European physician and surgeon Guglielmo da Saliceto (1210–1277):

> When I saw him lying with his intestines gashed, I was very worried, but I immediately caused hot wine to be brought (since there was no time to wait for something else) and warmed and bathed the intestines in this, while feces continued to come out from the various slashes. After I had washed them I drew the parts of the intestines together with a skinner's stitch, and put over the suture joining the lips of the wound a goodly quantity of [my adhesive] powder, which glued it together quickly; then after sewing them up I tried to reduce them but could not. So I took a razor and widened the wound to the necessary extent, and they went back in right away; then I united the parts of the *sifach* [peritoneum] and the external skin all together with a single stitch. I continued to watch over his treatment thereafter . . . and he recovered; eventually he had a wife and children and lived for a long time. (McVaugh 2006, 114–115)

In ancient India, surgeons used a more exotic cure, described in the *Susruta Samhita*:

> Large black ants should be applied even to the perforated intestines in such a case and their bodies should be separated from their heads after they had firmly bitten the perforated parts with their claws [i.e., jaws]. After that the intestines with the heads of the ants attached to them should be gently pushed back into the cavity and reinstated in their original situation therein. The bulged out intestines should be rinsed with grass, blood, and dust, washed with milk and lubricated with clarified butter and gently re-introduced into the cavity of the abdomen with the hand with its finger nails cleanly paired. The dried intestines should be washed with milk and lubricated with clarified butter before introducing it into their former and natural place in the abdomen. (Bhishagratna 1911, 272–273)

Using the vicelike grip of a large ant's mandibles to clamp a wound closed may sound shocking, but entomologists have confirmed that several species of ants might be used for this kind of procedure!

Head injuries also presented a particular challenge to the battlefield surgeon. If the surgeon suspected a fracture based on the injured soldier's symptoms, he needed to bare the skull (expanding the flesh wound if necessary) and scrape it to ascertain how deep it was. Paul of Aegina (ca. 625–ca. 690 C.E.) recommended that if the fracture was difficult to distinguish the surgeon should pour a solution of black writing ink onto the skull and scrape the bone on the following day when the fracture would be visible as a black line. In cases where the crack in the skull was deep and did not disappear with scraping, surgeons needed to use trephination, cutting the skull to remove any bone fragments that pressed upon the brain. The Hippocratic text, *On Wounds in the Head*, describes how to saw through the bone in detail, including the advice that, "while trephining, you should frequently take out the saw and plunge it into cold water to avoid heating the bone, for the saw gets heated by rotation, and by heating and drying the bone cauterizes it and makes more of the bone around the trephined part come away than was going to do" (Withington 1944b, 49).

The extraction of arrows would also have required specialized training and equipment. One Roman surgeon emphasized that soldiers should be told, "to put up with the arrows until they can have them removed by a person who can do so properly," because, "it can escape even an altogether experienced man that the point [of the arrow] is concealed" (Salazar 2000, 47–48). As he suggests, one of the real dangers in extracting arrows was if the shaft should come away leaving the arrowhead behind, making it difficult for the surgeon to find and remove. Otherwise, the surgeon needed to determine whether the arrow should be simply pulled out through the side it had entered or pushed through the body, perhaps making an incision on the other side of the body through which it could be extracted. The Islamic surgeon, Abu al-Qasim al-Zahrawi (fl. ca. 1000, known as Albucasis in the Latin West), described an especially difficult case he had treated.

> I once drew out an arrow from one of the officers of the State, that had struck him in the middle of the nose and was inclining a little to the right, and the whole arrow was buried. I was called to treat him three days after he had received the arrow wound; and I found the arrow wound very narrow. I explored it with a fine probe but did not find it; but the patient felt a pricking and a pain beneath the right ear, and I hoped that the pricking was due to the arrow. So I applied a poultice to the spot, a poultice with power to draw out and cause suppuration, desiring that the place should swell and that a sign to indicate the arrow should appear so that I could cut down upon it. But nothing happened at that place to indicate that the arrow had come through to there; so I persevered with poulticing it for many days; yet nothing fresh manifested itself and the wound healed up meanwhile, and the patient despaired for a time of its extraction. Then one day he felt the arrow inside his nose, and he told me of this; so for a number of days I applied a caustic medicine to the wound until it opened. I explored it, and felt the slim end of the arrow which is fastened to the shaft then I enlarged the opening of the wound by the use of the caustic until the tip of the arrow was plainly visible to me. About four months passed. Then when the wound was enlarged and I was able to introduce forceps into it I pulled on it and moved it, but it would not come out. And I went on skillfully and gently trying for it with various instruments until one day I caught hold of it with a pair of strong forceps . . . and drew it out; then dressed the wound. The medical men judged that the cartilage of the nose would not be restored, but I restored it and the wound healed up and the patient made a complete recovery nor did he suffer any harm. (Spink and Lewis 1973, 610–614)

Clearly, the extraction of arrows was not a simple task, requiring specialized tools, patience, and no doubt a great deal of pain for the patient!

In extreme cases, war wounds might necessitate the amputation of limbs. This might occur when a slashing wound had already nearly severed the limb, when crushed bones were too severely damaged to be set, or when gangrene set in, threatening to destroy the entire limb and claim the wounded soldier's life. The surgical manuals typically indicate that amputation was only done to remove lower joints; when gangrene had spread above the elbow or knee, one Islamic physician advised, "there is nothing of any avail in this case but to leave it, and for the patient to resign himself to death" (Savage-Smith 2000, 316). The operation entailed applying a ligature to the limb above and below the site to be cut then, following the operation, the wound would be cauterized and styptics would be applied to staunch bleeding. Evidence regarding the survival rate for this operation is mixed, but the risks were severe as another Islamic physician reported: "I once saw a group of thieves in the hospital whose hands and feet had been cut off. Their limbs became spasmodic because of the amputation, and not a single one of them escaped death" (Savage-Smith 2000, 316). On the other hand, the physician al-Zahrawi recorded examining a patient in Spain, who had previously amputated his own foot after it was infected with gangrene. When this man requested that the physician amputate his diseased hand, al-Zahrawi refused, fearing that the operation could lead to the patient's death; he later discovered that the patient had cut off the hand himself and recovered!

As the previous allusion to gangrene suggests, death from the initial wound was not all a soldier might need to worry about. Chances of infection were great and it is likely that more soldiers died from infected wounds than those who succumbed to injuries during the battle itself. Gangrene posed a significant threat, but so did other wound infections. Surgeons expected a degree of inflammation around the wound, which would typically be accompanied by fever, and suppuration. Depending upon how widely the inflammation spread or whether it exuded a "good" or "bad" pus, the surgeon stood ready to intervene as necessary with medicines or to drain off "bad" pus from abscesses around the wound. An account in the Edwin Smith papyrus offers an example of how an Egyptian *swnw* would approach postoperative care of a shoulder wound:

> You should say concerning him: "One having a gaping wound in his shoulder, its flesh being laid back and its sides separated, while he suffers with swelling (in) his shoulder blade. An ailment which I will treat." You should bind it with fresh meat the first day. If you find that wound open and its stitching loose, you should draw together for him its gash with two strips of linen over that gash; you should treat it afterward (with) grease, honey, (and) lint every day until he recovers. If you find a wound, its flesh laid back, its sides separated, in any member of a man, you should treat it according to these directions. If, however, you find that his flesh has developed inflammation from that wound which is in his shoulder, while that wound is inflamed, open, and its stitching loose,

you should lay your hand upon it. Should you find inflammation issu-
ing from the mouth of his wound at your touch, and secretions discharg-
ing therefrom are cool like *wenesh*-juice you should say concerning him:
"One having a gaping wound in his shoulder, it being inflamed, and he
continues to have fever from it. An ailment with which I will contend."
If, then you find that man continuing to have fever, while that wound is
inflamed, you should not bind it; you should moor (him) at his mooring
stakes [i.e. continue with a regular diet and do not administer any medi-
cines], until the period of his injury passes by. (Breasted 1930, 417–424)

Recovering from these kinds of injuries would be difficult in any circumstances, but for a soldier in an army on the march the onset of
wound infections would have frequently been fatal.

## DISEASE AND HUNGER IN WAR

One Egyptian text describes the life of a soldier on campaign:

He is called up for Syria. He may not rest. There are no clothes, no san-
dals. His march is uphill through mountains. He drinks water every
third day; it is smelly and tastes of salt. His body is ravaged by illness.
The enemy comes and life recedes from him. He is told, "Quick forward,
valiant soldier! Win for yourself a good name!" He does not know what
he is about. His body is weak, his legs fail him. If he leaps and joins the
deserters, all his people are imprisoned. He dies on the edge of the des-
ert, and there is none to perpetuate his name. (Archer, Ferris, Herwig,
and Travers 2002, 12)

Although it was likely written specifically to emphasize the inglorious
aspects of being a soldier, this account makes clear that military life
entailed far more than simply fighting in battles. Long marches with
little food or water and the ever-present threat of disease could exact a
far deadlier toll on an army than battles.

Epidemic diseases including smallpox, cholera, diphtheria, typhus,
dysentery, and numerous other febrile and diarrheal diseases regularly
afflicted armies in the premodern world, claiming many a soldier's
life. Indeed, diseases like the "bloody flux" (as dysentery was known)
were often endemic. Poor nutrition, contaminated water supplies,
inadequate camp sanitation, sleeping on cold or marshy ground, and
close quarters weakened soldiers' immune systems, ensuring that any
epidemic could spread swiftly through the ranks. And, nobody was
immune to these depredations; for example, the army of King Henry V
of England (1413–1422) suffered severely from dysentery throughout
his Agincourt campaign and the king himself finally died from the

bloody flux in 1422 at the young age of thirty-five, likely having contracted it while besieging the town of Meaux during a later campaign in France.

Early in the first century C.E., the Romans started to build hospitals (*valetudinaria*) in the permanent military forts on the frontiers of the Empire for the treatment of sick and wounded soldiers. These forts were typically many days behind the actual battle lines, so injured soldiers would be treated in the field, and the seriously injured would likely die before they could be transported back to the hospitals. However, the *valetudinaria* provided a space where wounded soldiers could receive post-operative care and soldiers afflicted with the inevitable camp diseases that followed armies could recuperate. A Roman hospital was typically constructed with the need to limit the spread of disease in mind. They were usually designed as a large rectangular building, having a main corridor running around the building with cubicles opening off of both sides where the patients could sleep away from draughts and noise. Additionally, the hospitals would have a large hall with good illumination that could serve as an operating room or reception area. Romans also made sure that the hospitals were supplied with plenty of fresh water and constructed sewers and latrines to remove waste. The staff of a Roman hospital typically included one or two doctors (*medici*), along with a range of other healthcare providers, including bandagers, students, and drug dispensers.

Frontier military garrisons during the Han dynasty (206 B.C.E.–220 C.E.) in China were similarly equipped with medical supplies and physicians. Each garrison was expected to maintain a careful register of troop illnesses like this one:

> Gao Zidang, private soldier of the 24th beacon unit, fell sick with headache on the seventh day of the fourth month and was unable to raise his four limbs; Zhou Liang, private soldier of Bingting beacon unit, fell sick and suffered cold damage on the fifth day of the fourth month; Jiang Tan, private soldier of the second beacon unit, fell sick on the sixth day of the fourth month and suffered swelling and fullness of the heart and belly; . . . Su Shang, private soldier of the thirty-seventh beacon unit, fell sick with arrow wounds to both flanks on the first day of the third month, and is slightly better; . . . Shangwu, private soldier of the thirty-first beacon unit, fell sick with headache on the eighth day of the fourth month, he had cold and heat, drank five doses of drug and has not yet recovered. (Guihua 2005, 91)

These somewhat monotonous records show that armies were susceptible to wounds, illness and disease even when not actively on campaign. Other records indicate that these garrisons were usually well supplied with the ingredients necessary to mix drugs to treat many different diseases including chronic coughs, diarrhea, "accumulation" in the heart and belly, "cold damage," and for "curing itching."

## SIEGE WARFARE

Warfare hit civilians especially hard. The *chevauchée*, a tactic of warfare employed during the European Middle Ages (and similar to the tactics of invading armies in general), employed mobile mounted soldiers to range across enemy territory and spread terror by burning crops and homes, stealing livestock, and killing peasants without mercy. Faced with these tactics, many peasants abandoned their farms in despair and fled into nearby woods to hide and wait for the army to pass. Other peasants might choose to flee and seek protection behind the walls of a nearby city.

Huddling behind the walls of a city may have provided protection against the immediate depredations of an invading army, but it brought entirely new problems if the army should choose to besiege the city: besieged cities were ideally suited for the spread of famine and disease. Cities facing a potential siege tried to gather a good supply of food and water behind their walls before the besieging army could arrive, with the intention of being able to defend the walls from the attackers and have sufficient resources to outlast the besiegers. This tactic often worked well since most armies could not carry enough food to be able to sustain a siege for more than a few weeks. In the end, it was not uncommon for both the besieging army and the besieged to grow hungry from lack of food.

Henry V's siege of Rouen, one of the wealthiest and most beautiful cities in France, gives some sense of what a siege may have been like. Learning of Henry's advance, the city stockpiled food, gathered from the surrounding countryside and destroyed any food they could not bring into the city so that there would be no easy supplies for Henry's army; once he arrived at Rouen at the end of July 1418 Henry needed to ship food across the English Channel and up the Seine River to feed his army. Rouen also received numerous refugees from the countryside, confident that its massive walls and stockpile of supplies would allow it to hold out against the attacking English army, at least until a French army could come and relieve the siege. No relieving army arrived, however, and Henry was able to import enough food to maintain his army, while supplies in the city were running low; by mid-October the people in the city were eating horseflesh and by December they were eating cats, dogs, rats, and even mice. Finally, the leaders of Rouen decided to expel the poor from the city to reduce the number of people they needed to feed; they drove more than 12,000 noncombatant refugees, including old men and nursing mothers, out of the city gates. King Henry did not wish to allow the city of Rouen to stretch their supplies and extend the siege in this way and refused to let the poor refugees pass beyond his siege lines, driving them back toward the city. When the leaders inside the city did not re-open the gates and allow the refugees to return, they were forced to huddle in the ditches outside the city walls where they were left to starve in the depths of winter. Many of Henry's English soldiers were horrified by the plight of the poor refugees now trapped beneath the walls and some even chose to share their food with them. One soldier described the scene in these terms:

> There one might see wandering here and there children of two or three years old begging for bread as their parents were dead. These wretched people had only sodden soil under them and they lay there crying for food—some starving to death, some unable to open their eyes no longer breathing, others cowering on their knees as thin as twigs. A woman was there clutching her dead child to her breast to warm it, and a child was sucking the breast of its dead mother. There one could easily count ten or twelve dead to one alive, who had died so quietly without call or cry as though they had died in their sleep. (Seward 1978, 176)

Conditions were little better within the city, and on New Years Eve the defenders sent envoys to parlay with Henry. The pleaded with the English king to allow the refugees to flee from beneath the walls, to which Henry replied, "I put them not there," and demanded that the city surrender. Finally, faced with famine behind the walls, even after having expelled 12,000 people from the city, Rouen agreed to surrender.

Along with famine, besieged cities might also succumb to an outbreak of epidemic disease. The Greek historian Thucydides documented the Spartan siege of the city of Athens during the Peloponnesian War (431–404 B.C.E.) where this was the case. Faced with a superior invading Spartan army, the Athenian leader Pericles (ca. 495–429 B.C.E.) advised that the people of Attica withdraw behind the walls of Athens and avoid a direct battle with the Spartans. He argued that since the Athenians would still have access to their harbor they would be able to resupply the city with food by sea, while the Spartan army would run out of food and be forced to withdraw. At first, the plan seemed sound, but an epidemic broke out within the city and many people, including

Pericles, died. Thucydides explains that the calamity of the disease was aggravated by the overcrowding behind the walls and that the high mortality and confines of the city meant that the Athenians were unable to observe the usual burial customs. Seeing the smoke from the funeral pyres and learning of the spread of plague within the city, the Spartans finally withdrew, fearing that they might become infected, but this was no victory for Athens.

The dangers of famine and disease aside, defenders faced many other threats during a siege. Attacking armies often used powerful siege engines (like catapults and trebuchets) to try to batter down the walls or throw large stones into the city. Perhaps the most immediate concern for defenders was when their enemies used these devices to throw incendiary devices over the walls to spread fires, an extreme danger in any premodern city. It was also common for armies to catapult dead and diseased animals, and even the severed heads and limbs of captured enemies, into cities. These actions served the twofold purpose of inciting fear within the city and also of spreading disease—an early form of biological warfare.

# CHAPTER 12

# Institutions and Health

Beyond the work of doctors treating individual patients, larger institutions such as charitable groups, religious organizations (e.g., churches and monasteries), and governments (both locally and on a national level) engaged in funding large-scale programs for attending to the health and welfare of the general populace. The activities of these institutions could take the form of building projects that would promote sanitation and public health or fund the construction and maintenance of hospitals that could provide charitable care to the poor. In other cases, the sanction and support of civil and religious authorities was necessary to regulate medical activities and to encourage certain forms of medically related research, especially that related to the study of human anatomy. These activities sponsored by the state or by religious organizations reflected ideals of the general populace and general attitudes about how best to see to the health needs of the larger population. Nonetheless, we should also recognize that many of these state or religiously sponsored activities were not necessarily concerned with preventative medicine and medical research, for the same reasons as we may expect today; indeed, they were often motivated by goals that were not necessarily associated with an interest in providing health.

## GOVERNMENTAL AND RELIGIOUS INSTITUTIONS IN MESOPOTAMIA AND EGYPT

### Irrigation Systems

One of the most significant needs of early civilizations, especially those in the relatively dry climates of Mesopotamia and Egypt, was to ensure a sufficient supply of water to sustain crops that would feed the growing urban populations. This task required the development of irrigation systems that could deliver water to crops in the right amounts at the right times. Furthermore, irrigation systems needed to be designed that could reduce the threat of flooding and that could store water for use during the dry season. Evidence reveals that irrigation systems were being built in both Mesopotamia and Egypt as early as the sixth millennium B.C.E., when individual farmers were likely able to take measures to see to their own water needs. As the civilizations grew, however, the need to develop more complex irrigation systems often required large investments in labor and capital, which might in turn have necessitated increased governmental oversight to fund and coordinate their construction.

The Nile River was the source of life in ancient Egypt. It receives no tributaries during its course through Egypt, and it therefore provides the only regular source of fresh water in the region. Fortunately for the inhabitants of ancient Egypt, the flow of the Nile is exceedingly predictable, beginning in June with the snowmelt in the highlands of Africa, rising to a peak in late September or early October and then receding by the end of November. This regularity allowed ancient Egyptians to plan for one crop season per year, which would be planted in the soil watered by the floods. They dug simple canals that would reach to the high point of the Nile's flood, with sluices at their mouths that could regulate how much water was directed from the river into the fields. Water would be left in the fields for months to saturate the ground thoroughly and then would be drained off through another system of canals prior to planting the crops. By 1500 B.C.E., the Egyptians were making use of a *shadouf*, a simple tool composed of a long pole suspended in the middle by braces with a weight on one end and a bucket on another, which could be used to raise water from a lower level to canals at a higher level, further enhancing the irrigation system.

The regularity of the flooding meant that the ancient Egyptians were not especially concerned with developing systems for water storage since the summer floods provided sufficient water for a crop season. However, they were always concerned with determining how high the river would reach in its flood since this dictated how far to dig the canals. For this reason they built a series of "nilometers," spaced along the river, which allowed them to monitor the height of the Nile at various points and thus predict with some accuracy the high water mark. Furthermore, records in palaces and temples recorded the level reached by the flood each year to aid in these predictions. Aside from these efforts at prediction, the Egyptian irrigation systems were fairly simple and did not require a vast number of laborers to build and maintain, suggesting that they were likely designed and built at a local level, without the intervention of the central government. Indeed, the fact that no written laws concerning water regulation exist in the legal codes of ancient Egypt suggests that the water management system was not complex or contentious enough to require significant governmental intervention.

Mesopotamia, the land between the Tigris and Euphrates rivers, faced very different conditions from Egypt. Whereas the flooding of the Nile was gentle and predictable from year-to-year, the Tigris and Euphrates rivers were far less regular and were liable to run dry or bring sudden flash floods. Faced with these concerns, the Mesopotamians needed to develop an irrigation system that would protect against sudden floods and that could create areas for water storage. Furthermore, the Mesopotamian irrigation systems were more prone to the danger of salination (the accumulation of salts in the soil caused by repeated irrigation) than in Egypt. Increased soil salinity would prevent crops from growing in the fields (sometimes for one hundred years or more) and Mesopotamian history records several salinity crises that necessitated the abandonment of previously arable land. As might be expected, the unpredictable supply of water prompted numerous disputes over water rights, as attested in the surviving legal records.

The more significant technical challenges of designing and coordinating an irrigation system and the prevalence of legal disputes over water, required greater centralized governmental oversight than in Egypt. Whereas individual farmers or local communities might coordinate to build and maintain their irrigation systems in Egypt, in Mesopotamia city-states passed laws requiring farmers to contribute labor to build and maintain canals and also dictated where canals would be built. Perhaps the earliest example of this process is from around 2400 B.C.E. under the king Entemenak of Girsu. The city-states of Girsu and Umma along the Euphrates had disputed water rights and Umma, upstream of Girsu, had regularly breached canals dug by the people of Girsu to irrigate their crops. In order to provide water for Girsu, Entemenak oversaw the digging of a vast canal to the Tigris

River that was thereafter able to provide irrigation for the city's fields; by about 1700 B.C.E., this canal was so large and important that it was known simply as "the Tigris." Similarly, the Assyrian ruler, Sennacherib (704–681 B.C.E.), oversaw the construction of a massive irrigation system and also built a massive aqueduct to supply water to his capital city of Nineveh. Reflecting the extreme importance of irrigation in Mesopotamian society, Sennacherib boasted that it was he

> who digs canals, opens irrigated fields, and makes irrigation ditches murmur (with water); who established prosperity and abundance in the wide crop-lands of Assyria; who put irrigation water in the fields of Assyria where, from days of old, no one had seen, no one had known, those who preceded me had not made, canals and irrigation in Assyria. (Russell 1987, 535)

These activities make clear the important role of kings and the state in developing irrigation systems in ancient Mesopotamia.

### Embalming in Ancient Egypt and Knowledge of the Body

Governmental and religious institutions in ancient Egypt supported conditions that allowed for the opening of the body, although this was not usually done for the purposes of gaining medical or scientific knowledge. Embalmers in ancient Egypt displayed extensive technical expertise in opening the body and preparing it for mummification. They were able to remove internal organs through relatively small incisions, including the brain, which was extracted through the nose after perforating the ethmoid bone. The lungs, stomach, liver, and intestines would then be transferred to four separate canopic jars; the heart, deemed the site of intelligence in the body, was not removed. The body cavity would then be washed out with oils and preserving fluids, stuffed with straw and linen, and the incisions would be covered (in one mummy the incision was closed with sutures). Finally, the body would be covered in natron, a natural salt, which was also put into the cavities, and left to dry out for roughly forty days before being wrapped.

These procedures attest to the embalmers' general knowledge of major anatomical structures and of methods of preservation. It is not clear, however, whether the embalmers passed their anatomical skills to doctors. Herodotus (ca. 484–ca. 425 B.C.E.), a Greek historian, who wrote extensively about the beliefs and practices of other cultures, observed that in his time the embalmers were regarded as ritually unclean and were thus unlikely to have communicated extensively with doctors, or that surgeons would have been able to practice their skills by helping to prepare mummies. Thus, although embalmers fulfilled an important state-sponsored function, the anatomical knowledge they gleaned was likely of little value to medical practitioners.

## INSTITUTIONAL SUPPORT FOR HEALTH AND MEDICINE IN ANCIENT GREECE AND ROME

### The Museum and the Library in Alexandria, Egypt

After the death of Alexander the Great (356–323 B.C.E.), his vast territories were divided up among his leading generals. One of his Greek generals, Ptolemy, seized control of Egypt and thenceforth his family ruled as the pharaohs, establishing a Greek dynasty in the country that ended with the death of queen Cleopatra VII (69–30 B.C.E.) and the Roman conquest in 30 B.C.E. The city of Alexandria served as the capital city of the Ptolemies and grew to be one of the most populous cities in the ancient world. The early Ptolemies were great patrons of the arts and sciences. Perhaps their most important activities in this regard were the foundation of the Museum (a temple of the Muses) as a philosophical school like Plato's Academy and their willingness to provide financial support to any scholars willing to live and work there. They also built the Alexandrian Library, associated with the Museum, in which they gathered written works on all subjects of learning. Whenever scholars arrived in Alexandria their scrolls would be examined and if they contained texts not already in the Library, they would be confiscated and copied by scribes, and then the copy would be returned to the owner while the original would be added to the collection. In this way, the Library grew to become the greatest library of the ancient world. Together, the Museum and the Library served to make Alexandria the center of learning in the Mediterranean for several centuries.

The Ptolemaic patronage of scholarship and research extended to providing support for the study of human anatomy through dissection and possibly vivisection. Although such activities would likely have been prevented in the rest of the Greek world due to strict religious taboos against handling dead bodies, two medical researchers at Alexandria are especially associated with the study of human anatomy: Herophilus (335–280 B.C.E.) and Erasistratus (304–250 B.C.E.). Both men were said to have dissected the bodies of criminals, who were provided by the authority of the government, for the purposes of medical research; some ancient accounts even suggest that Herophilus and Erasistratus vivisected criminals, that is, dissected them while they were still alive! In his later works on human anatomy Galen of Pergamum (129–ca. 216 C.E.) refers to the anatomical discoveries of Erasistratus and Herophilus on several occasions, but by his time it appears that the cultural taboos against cutting dead bodies had been reasserted; indeed, it is unlikely that Galen ever dissected human bodies. Nonetheless, for a brief period of time under the institutional support provided by Ptolemaic patronage, the study of human anatomy through the dissection of human bodies was made possible in the ancient world.

### Roman Engineering: Aqueducts and Sewage Systems

Sextus Julius Frontinus (ca. 40–104 C.E.) served in the Roman army and later as the Provincial Governor in Britain before being appointed the Water Commissioner for Rome. He wrote about the responsibilities of this position in his *De aquis urbis Romae* (*On the Aqueducts of the City of Rome*), which provides many details of the water supply of ancient Rome and in which he boasts that his work in this regard improved the health of the city. According to Frontinus, Roman inhabitants originally obtained their water from the Tiber River or from private wells. However, in the year 312 B.C.E. the consul, Appius Claudius Crassus, who had overseen the construction of the great road, known as the Appian Way, which connected southern Italy to Rome, built an aqueduct to bring fresh water to the city from springs in the Alban hills. Other aqueducts were built so that by the first century C.E., Rome was supplied with fresh water by means of nine aqueducts, with different systems for supplying drinking water and water for use in gardens or industry. The Roman system of aqueducts was designed to produce a constant gravitational flow of water, with settling tanks (*piscinae*) along that line that served to trap the silt and could be used to raise the water to higher elevations. Water flowed continuously from the aqueducts to a number of public fountains in the city, providing fresh water to inhabitants, and the overflow from the fountains was allowed to wash the streets and flush the sewers.

By the first century C.E., the maintenance of the aqueducts was a fulltime job and a position of *curator aquarum* (procurator of the water supply) of consular rank was created with two assistants of senatorial rank to oversee this work. The emperor Augustus (r. 27 B.C.E.–14 C.E.) bequeathed 240 skilled slaves to the city for the purpose of caring for the water supply systems and this number was augmented by an additional 460 slaves bequeathed by the emperor Claudius (r. 41–54 C.E.), attesting to the amount of labor involved and the value given to this work by the imperial leaders. It was in his role as the procurator of the water supply that Frontinus came to write his book on the aqueducts of Rome. He describes their construction and the difficulties faced by those in his position. One problem in particular was the illegal siphoning of water from the system:

> My investigations show that they [employees of the water Catchment Board responsible for maintaining the water supply] have been diverting water from public conduits for private use. There is also a significant number of landowners tapping the conduits that by-pass their property. As a result, the public supply is brought to a standstill by private citizens just to water their gardens ... I found irrigated fields, shops, garrets even, and every house of ill repute in Rome, with fixtures to ensure constant running water. (Amulree 1973, 245)

No wonder the Romans needed to appoint so many officials to supervise the water supply systems!

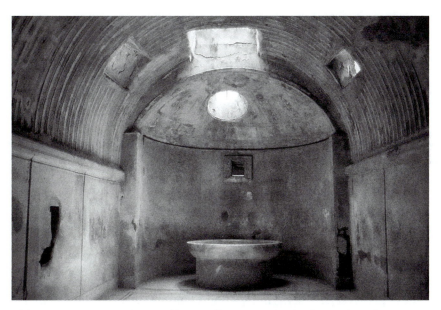

This is the interior of the *caldarium* (hot water bath) located in the Forum Baths of Pompeii, Italy. The central marble *labrum* (basin) was filled with colder water for those who became too hot. Hot water was heated in an underground furnace and directed through pipes into the appropriate rooms. Other rooms in the bath house would contain a warm water pool (*tepidarium*) and a cold water pool (*frigidarium*). Hot air was often channeled through empty space under the floors to heat the floor tiles. Large bathing houses might also contain an exercise area (*palaestra*). (Allan T. Kohl/Art Images for College Teaching)

The Romans were concerned with individual hygiene and starting in the second century C.E., they built public baths (*thermae*), often at the expense of Rome's richest citizens and emperors, making them available to the poorest Romans. These bathhouses usually had furnaces for heating water and they even engineered methods for sending hot air under the floors to provide a form of central heating to the rooms. They would typically have many different rooms for cold baths (*frigidarium*) and hot baths (*caldarium*), with changing rooms for men and women and rooms where people could contract the services of barbers and masseuses. Although people went to them for the purpose of hygiene and for their health, the bathhouses were in many ways the center of urban life and people would regularly meet in them to socialize at the end of the day. One Roman, whose apartment was located above one such establishment, complained of the noise that rose from the many bathers, people exercising before their baths, and all of the food vendors, barbers, and others, hawking their wares to the bathhouse clientele.

One of the other great marvels of Roman engineering was their sewer system. The *Cloaca Maxima*, the main conduit of the Roman sewage system running from the Forum to the Tiber River, dates to around the sixth century C.E., when it was constructed to drain local marshes. In the following years, a network of conduits was connected to it and it served to drain storm water and sewage. The government also paid for the construction of public latrines and cesspits that were emptied at various times; a census reveals that there were roughly 150 public latrines in Rome during the reign of Emperor Constantine (r. 306–337 C.E.). Some of these latrines were free, but some charged a small fee. Romans did not have toilet paper, but would often supply each bathroom with a sponge on a stick for the use of its patrons that could be rinsed out between uses in a bowl of water. The maintenance and care of the sewer system was also undertaken by the state, and governmental officials were appointed to oversee these projects.

## INSTITUTIONAL MEDICINE IN ANCIENT INDIA

During the reign of King Ashoka (ca. 273–232 B.C.E.), the third king of the Mauryan age, centralized royal administration was increasingly exerted over the empire and the government became greatly involved in the spread of medical care, among other things, to the general population in India. At the start of his reign, King Ashoka was renowned for his military conquests and cruelty. He famously had many of his brothers murdered in his rise to power and later maintained an extensive prison filled with a wide range of torture devices, which he employed upon criminals and enemies. About eight years into his reign, however, Ashoka witnessed the aftermath of a war he had waged, the loss of life and social turmoil that it caused, and was deeply affected by the experience. As a result, he resolved to abandon his program of conquest and dedicate the remainder of his life to applying Buddhist principles to the administration of his territories. He outlined his new principles in a series of edicts carved on stone pillars that were distributed throughout his empire (they have been found in over thirty sites within India, Nepal, Pakistan, and Afghanistan). In the Rock Edicts, Ashoka apologized for the suffering his wars had caused and declared that he would look upon his subjects as his children and make their welfare his main concern in the future.

Many of the edicts are aimed at enacting judicial reforms, but also encouraged the practice of religion (he promoted Buddhism but sought the protection of all religions and encouraged harmony between them) and moral reforms. To ensure that his reforms were carried out, he traveled the empire on inspection tours and he expected his officials to do likewise. Many edicts indicate that Ashoka believed the state should have an important role in fostering the provision of healthcare to his people; the second rock edict in particular proclaims that everywhere within his empire the state should make provision for the medical care of humans and animals. According to the edicts, the state should see to the importation or cultivation of medicinal herbs and fruits in all parts of the empire, as well as dig wells for fresh water along main roads, and plant groves of trees along the roads to provide shade for humans and animals. These public works activities aimed at the provision of healthcare for his subjects encouraged the idea in India that the care of the sick should be a social responsibility.

Under later Mauryan kings, the state developed a bureau dedicated to directing the settlement of uncultivated land and to controlling the distribution of water. Land and water were regarded as properties of the king, and the state developed irrigation canals and water storage cisterns and demanded revenues in the form of taxes and rents for such services. These state funded irrigation projects provided water for agriculture and also for the growing cities throughout the empire. Although centralized government control was not always as powerful after the death of Ashoka, in later centuries, kings continued to emphasize the importance of public irrigation projects dedicated to maintaining the economic vitality of the state and the welfare of the people. Specialized hydraulic engineers were charged with the construction and maintenance of irrigation and water storage facilities, and it appears that treatises on the science of hydrology circulated widely in south India by the fourteenth century C.E., These texts provided information on the different kinds of irrigation canals, and how and where to dig wells and construct storage cisterns. They also emphasized the importance of planting trees along the banks of canals to arrest soil erosion and breaches due to flooding. In other parts of India, hydraulic engineers also built irrigation works on a massive scale, damming rivers and creating large artificial lakes to serve as water reservoirs, many of which still exist today. One of these reservoirs, the Colagangam constructed under Rajendra I (r. 1012–1044), was sixteen miles long.

Ashoka also generously supported the development of Buddhist monastic communities (*sanghas*). Buddhist monasteries had played a significant role in the development of medicine in India since the fifth century B.C.E., especially in regards to the rise of the written medical tradition and as centers of medical education. Although most often they offered a refuge for travelers, they also came to serve as important institutions for the provision of healthcare. The *Caraka Samhita* describes such early medical institutions, "halls for health" or what we might consider hospitals, which were dedicated to providing care to the sick, emphasizing that in the interests of patients the hospital should be constructed, "out of the path of smoke, sunlight, water, or dust, as well as unwanted noise, feelings, tastes, sights, and smells. It should have a water supply, pestle and mortar, lavatory, bathing area, and a kitchen" (Wujastyk 2003, 36). In addition to the general construction of the halls for health, the author of the *Caraka* describes the personnel, tools, and medicines with which it should be equipped. He intended that these halls be furnished so as to treat not only a patient's physical ailments, but also maintain her emotional and mental health by providing a serene and pleasant environment. To this end, attendants were expected to be skilled at medicine, but also able to sing, play musical instruments, recite verses, and tell stories to entertain the sick. Although it represents an idealized picture of what an Indian hospital might look like, it does reflect the early appearance of health care institutions in the Indian subcontinent.

## HEALTH AND THE STATE IN CHINA

The state played an especially important role in the regulation of health from an early point in Chinese history. As we have seen in other chapters, the central Chinese government took control over medical education as early as the second century B.C.E., creating imperial universities and administering qualifying examinations for medical students. Likewise, the state took responsibility for the standardization of pharmacopeias and other medical texts by the seventh century C.E. and established state run pharmaceutical dispensaries that were charged with overseeing the manufacture and sale of drugs to ensure their quality throughout the empire. Through these efforts, the central imperial government in China took an active role in regulating the provision of medical care that was not matched in other premodern societies.

The earliest institutions providing charitable healthcare in China were those associated with Buddhist monasteries, as in India. During the Tang dynasty (618–907 C.E.), the state gradually assumed control over the Buddhist healthcare institutions; in the eighth century state run orphanages and infirmaries for the destitute were established and then in the mid-ninth century Buddhist monasteries and lands were nationalized, and the revenues from those properties were used to fund charitable hospitals. The emperors of the Song dynasty (960–1279 C.E.) continued to establish free hospitals for the care of the sick poor in major cities in the empire. These state run charitable institutions were expensive, however, and by the late Ming dynasty (ca. 1500–1644) emperors ceased to sponsor these medical services, and private charities stepped in to pay for hospitals for the poor.

Increasing urbanization during the Song period also encouraged state sponsorship of a number of other activities that provided for the general health and welfare of city dwellers. In particular, the authorities in the Song dynasty implemented measures to enhance public health and hygiene in cities. In the capital city of Hangchow in the thirteenth century C.E., for example, numerous canals were dug to allow for transportation and irrigation in and around the city. Furthermore, an artificial lake was created and carefully maintained to serve as a reservoir for pure drinking water, and earthenware conduits were built to bring fresh water from the lake into the city. Public authorities also paid for street sweepers and garbage removal (garbage was removed by boats on the canals and left on wasteland outside the city), and groups of nightsoil collectors gathered waste from cesspools, which was either taken from the city or used as fertilizer in gardens and vegetable plots. By comparison with European cities in this period, Hangchow was a very clean city, a fact that Marco Polo commented on in some amazement, noting that travelers, "both on horseback and on foot [can walk] through all the lands of it without soiling the feet" (Wright 1962, 42). Although these public efforts to maintain the city's cleanliness were not necessarily taken strictly for the purposes of maintaining health in the city, they would have served an important role in reducing the risk of epidemic disease.

## HOSPITALS IN THE ISLAMIC WORLD
## AND MEDIEVAL EUROPE

In the Islamic world, the most visible institution dedicated to the provision of healthcare was the hospital. The earliest Islamic hospitals emerged in the late eighth or early ninth century in Iraq and were modeled on the Nestorian Christian hospices, charitable institutions that provided shelter to travelers and the poor and also assumed the task of providing medical care to the infirm. However, the Islamic hospitals, or *bimaristans* as they were called, increasingly took on a more specifically medical function in Islamic society than had been the case in the Christian hospices; whereas Christian hospices were typically governed by monks and served a religious function, the Islamic hospitals were most often overseen by elite physicians and were secular in character.

The *bimaristans* were typically founded by acts of royal patronage to provide free medical care to the poor and were often symbols of the charity and prestige of the ruler. By the twelfth century, any large Islamic town in the East or North Africa would have a hospital, making them significant medical institutions in Islam. Despite their wide geographic distribution, however, their influence as a source of medical relief was limited; people living in the countryside did not have access to hospital care, and hospitals could only receive a small number of patients in comparison to the size of the urban populations they served.

Hospitals made their greatest impact in the Islamic world, therefore, not as sites of treatment, but rather as centers for the dissemination of learned medicine. *Bimaristans* attracted the elite physicians from the Islamic world, such as Abu Bakr Muhammad ibn Zakariya al-Razi (d. ca. 925, known as Rhazes in the Latin West), and positions in the hospitals would provide markers of prestige and financial security. Physicians would visit and treat patients in the hospitals in addition to maintaining their own private clients (al-Razi, for example, counted many high-ranking officials among his private patients). Many of the physicians drawn to the hospitals were also scholars involved in the translation of ancient Greek and also Ayurvedic medical texts, and many wrote their own books on medicine. In this way, the hospitals developed renown as centers for medical learning and attracted students from all over the Islamic world. Indeed, it appears that many hospitals had libraries and larger rooms set aside as lecture halls, and students would often accompany the physicians on their rounds.

In addition to their role in disseminating learned medical knowledge, the *bimaristans* were complex institutions, prepared to meet a variety of medical needs. Hospital staffs included numerous physicians, surgeons, oculists, bone-setters, and pharmacists, as well as orderlies charged with providing basic care and administrators who were not involved in treating patients, but would oversee the general functioning of the hospital. Hospitals were divided into a number of wards, reserved for people suffering from different conditions (e.g., wings were set aside for the mentally ill, those with eye ailments, those recovering from surgery, patients with specific gastrointestinal disorders, etc.), with separate halls for male and female patients. Furthermore, they had rooms for the pharmacy as well as kitchens, living quarters for the staff, latrines and storage areas. These divisions allowed hospitals to accommodate a range of conditions, from those who might require only brief stays to those who would need more long-term medical care.

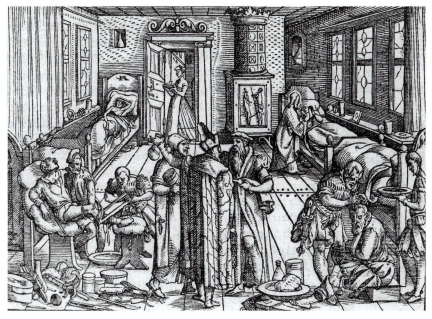

This is a European hospital scene from around 1565, which emphasizes both the medical and religious goals of hospitals. It shows patients in bed and receiving medical care. In the foreground, three physicians with their backs to the patients debate the significance of the signs they see in the urine flask, which one of them holds. Meanwhile, surgeons are actively engaged in treating patients, performing an amputation on the left and a trephination on the right. A nurse also appears through a doorway bringing food. In the background, Christ (recognized by his halo) cares for a sick patient. This image was clearly intended to aggrandize the work of surgeons over physicians; surgeons, like Christ, are seen actively caring for patients, while the physicians are depicted as being more interested in theoretical debates than treating the sick. (Wellcome Library, London)

By contrast, hospitals in Western Europe during the Middle Ages continued to provide primarily religious aid and shelter for the poor and for pilgrims; medical assistance was often only a secondary concern. Indeed, many medieval European hospitals banned those suffering from fever, plague, or other contagious diseases for fear of spreading such afflictions to other patients and most did not have permanent physicians on staff, although some of the religious leaders who staffed hospitals had medical knowledge. Only during the later medieval period did some European hospitals increasingly start to set aside beds specifically for the sick poor and maintain physicians on staff, but even then the care was provided within a religious context, and hospitals did not become the centers of education that they were in the Islamic world. Even the leprosaria, special houses founded to provide aid to lepers, did not serve a primarily medical function, but rather aimed to provide charitable assistance to those deprived of shelter and livelihood as a result of their condition. Many urban hospitals, like the Hôtel-Dieu in Paris, from the mid-thirteenth century onward maintained special wards for pregnant women who had nowhere to live, or who wished to give birth in secret, and some even kept a midwife on staff, but again the charitable assistance was as much aimed at preventing infanticide in cases where women might wish to hide their sexual sins or where they could not afford to raise a child as it was at providing medical care.

## THE BLACK DEATH AND PUBLIC HEALTH IN MEDIEVAL EUROPE

The arrival of the Black Death in Europe in 1348 galvanized the interest of civic authorities in developing state run public health efforts. Initially, some towns, especially in Italy, established temporary committees to coordinate public health responses to the spread of the plague, which included isolating those infected with the disease, or evicting them from the city, imposing quarantines, and even outright banning refugees arriving from plague infested areas. Such measures required the administrative and financial support of the government; doctors alone would not have had the authority or power to enforce these regulations. By 1400, many towns had established permanent health boards that were composed of lay officials who were supported by medical advisers.

Health boards continued to enact and enforce quarantines and to close borders, but increasingly took additional actions to curb the spread of epidemic diseases. Cleaning the city to prevent the collection of materials that might produce the harmful airs, or miasmas, thought to spread disease became one of the main responsibilities of the health boards. Thus, in addition to seeing to the removal of sewage, health boards passed regulations requiring butchers, tanners, and other industries known for producing waste that could rot and produce foul smelling miasmas to dispose of their wastes in appropriate ways. In some cases, they also claimed the right to inspect the quality of meats, wine, and fish in the market for the good of the city.

In a perhaps more sinister role, health boards in some cities also created regulations to control the behavior of those deemed dangerous. Prostitutes were frequent targets of public health officials, who viewed them as a significant cause of the spread of infection. Likewise, beggars, "ruffians," and "loafers," were also viewed as potential carriers of plague. As a result, public health regulations often targeted these socially undesirable individuals under the guise of combating the spread of plague. In Venice, we find the following regulations, for example:

> Just as was done with prostitutes, it is necessary that male and female ruffians who are in the city be known to all, because they are the source of many evils. That is, others are persuaded by their example to live in their disgraceful fashion. So the [Venetian health board] by the power given them by the senate, have deliberated and decided that all these ruffians who are staying in the city must wear the color yellow. Thus they will be recognized by everyone. Violators will be whipped from San Marco to the Rialto, and then banished forever from the territory. (Carmichael 1986, 125)

Clearly, health boards acquired a wide-reaching authority to exert its influence on many areas of civic life.

# CHAPTER 13

# Healing and the Arts

## ENCOUNTERS WITH THE DOCTOR IN ART AND LITERATURE

Although it is not uncommon today for people to dismiss the practices of premodern medicine as superstitious and as having little more than a placebo effect at best, it is important to recognize that healers were often portrayed positively in art and literature across cultures in the premodern world. Some portrayals depict examples of the idealized or miraculous healer, serving as a model that average doctors might be expected to emulate, while others illustrate the more mundane, even messy aspects of medical practice. Considered together, these stories and visual depictions of healers provide useful insight into the status of healers in society, the general level of confidence in their curative abilities, and typical complaints about their failings.

In some cases, physicians were portrayed as having extraordinary, even miraculous, healing powers. One widely circulated legend in medieval Europe told of the medical activities of the brothers Cosmas and Damian, Christian physicians of the third century C.E. According to the legend, the brothers were learned in the art of medicine and were renowned for their willingness to treat patients, without accepting any reward for their services, symbolizing their Christian charity. The story most often told about Cosmas and Damian, which was the subject of many paintings in medieval and Renaissance Europe, recounts how they successfully transplanted the limb of a dead Ethiopian onto a white patient whose own cancerous leg they had removed. In conjunction with their charitable healing, this and other miraculous cures attributed to the brothers provided evidence of their sanctity and, after their martyrdom, they were recognized as the patron saints of physicians and surgeons throughout Europe. This story emblematizes a belief in the close connection between healing and faith in Christian culture and offers a model for the ideal Christian physician, trained in naturalistic medicine and motivated by religious piety to apply his knowledge charitably.

In China, legends about the physician Hua Tuo (ca. 145–208 C.E.) offer a similar account of a selfless healer, who could bring about spectacular cures by means of naturalistic medicine. According to stories, Hua Tuo turned down offers from eminent figures to assume a more lucrative career in government service, choosing rather to travel in the provinces curing peasants and seeking medical knowledge. He gained such renown for his medical skills (especially in acupuncture and surgery), however, that Cao Cao, ruler of a kingdom in northern China, demanded that Hua Tuo come to court and serve as his personal physician to treat his chronic headaches. Hua Tuo came and through the use of acupuncture alleviated the king's headaches, but he refused to remain at court, intending rather to return to his work in the provinces, and out of spite Cao Cao had him killed. The legends say that while in prison awaiting execution Hua Tuo wrote down his medical techniques, including his recipe for *mafeisan* (an anesthetic powder he used during surgery), but, "when Hua Tuo was about to be executed, he brought out a scroll with writing on it and handed it over to the jailer, saying, 'This can preserve people's lives.' Fearful of the law, the prison subaltern would not accept it, nor did Hua Tuo force it upon him. Instead, he asked for a fire in which he burned the scroll" (Mair 1994, 694). The loss of Hua Tuo's contribution to medical knowledge was regretted ever after.

More mundane physicians were depicted in art and literature as having mastered an extensive theoretical knowledge about the body and disease that was increasingly embedded in a sophisticated textual tradition. The mastery of this text-based knowledge distinguished the learned physicians from the wide range of other healers, whose knowledge of healing was grounded in empirical learning and craft practice with little emphasis on theoretical medicine. Therefore, physicians were often portrayed in close association with their books, or in the act of teaching students (see illustrations on pp. 6 and 180). Physicians were also portrayed in the act of diagnosis, taking the pulse, or studying the patient's urine. Successful use of these diagnostic techniques was supposed to require extensive textual training and many texts were written about them. Some of the texts even included illustrations of "urine wheels," showing the different colors of urine a physician may encounter and explaining which disease they may portend; these are similar to the pages of illustrations of tongues common in Chinese medical literature, which explain how to recognize signs of disease by examining the tongue. Indeed, the examination of urines came to be so closely associated with textual medical training that the urine flask came to be the symbol of scientific medicine in the European Middle Ages, similar to how the stethoscope and white lab coat are symbols of scientific medicine in the West today (see illustration on p. 217).

Healers were also often depicted in art in the act of mixing medicines or treating patients. Certain practices, as with the portrayal of diagnostic techniques, were often associated with those physicians trained in the textual medical tradition. For example, the application of moxibustion and acupuncture in China required significant training, and those depicted doing so would likely have been learned physicians (see illustration on p. 150). In other cases, healers might be shown in the act of surgery or with their surgical tools. Surgical skill was often highly regarded in Greek and Roman art and literature. In the *Iliad*, for example, when Menelaus was injured by an arrow, the soldiers immediately found one warrior, Machaon, the son of Asclepius, known for his surgical skills: "the god-sent healer reached the captain's side and quickly drew the shaft from his buckled belt—he pulled it clear, the sharp barbs broke back. . . . When he saw the wound where the tearing arrow hit, he sucked out the blood and deftly applied the healing salves that Chiron, friend of Asclepius, gave his father long ago" (Fagles 1990, 152). Greek and Roman doctors are similarly depicted in art engaged in surgical operations (see illustration on p. 142). By contrast, in China and medieval Europe, surgery was usually considered the province of lower status craftsmen and avoided by physicians. Indeed, in the artwork of the medieval West, it was not uncommon to see physicians portrayed as being so closely associated with the symbols of their textual training that they appeared uninterested in the actual task of treating patients! Surgeons and barber-surgeons, on the other hand, were often shown engaging in treating patients by performing surgical operations, letting blood, and cupping (healers were often shown with their cupping flasks), a stark contrast to images of physicians with their books and urine flasks, engaging in theoretical debates while their patients suffered quietly in the background! (see illustrations on pp. 157, 188, and 217).

In the general prologue to his *Canterbury Tales*, Geoffrey Chaucer (ca. 1343–1400) offers a typical portrait of the physician in medieval culture—one that may have seemed familiar in most of the cultures we have examined. Chaucer praises his "doctor of physic" for his deep knowledge of astrology and the written medical tradition:

> Nowhere in all the world was one to match him
> Where medicine was concerned, or surgery;
> Being well grounded in astrology
> He'd watch his patient with the utmost care
> Until he'd found a favorable hour,
> By means of astrology, to give treatment.
> Skilled to pick out the astrologic moment
> For charms and talismans to aid the patient,
> He knew the cause of every malady,
> If it were "hot" or "cold" or "moist" or "dry,"
> And where it came from, and from which humor.
> He was a really fine practitioner.
> . . .
> Well-read was he in Asclepius,
> In Dioscorides, and in Rufus,
> Ancient Hippocrates, Hali, and Galen,
> Avicenna, Rhazes, and Serapion,
> Averroës, Damascenus, Constantine,
> Bernard, and Gilbertus, and Gaddesden. (Wright 1985, 11–12)

Chaucer, a dedicated satirist, did not raise doubts about the efficacy of the physician's cures, however, and did not portray him as being too in love with theory to treat patients; indeed, he notes that the good doctor regularly attended the sick during the Black Death. From where did his doctor's motivation to treat the sick come? Not from a pious desire to treat the poor, such as displayed by Cosmas and Damian and Hua Tuo (indeed, Chaucer's physician "read but little in the Bible"), but rather because he was able to earn such high fees from those he treated, as Chaucer notes: "In medicine gold is the best cordial. So it was gold that he loved best of all" (Wright 1985, 11–12). Greed motivated the physician even more than love of theory!

## THE BODY IN MEDICAL ART

Medical texts in China and the medieval West often include a number of medical illustrations, revealing the importance of the visual representation of the medical body in both cultures. Sanskrit medical texts from the Ayurvedic tradition in premodern India, by contrast, were normally not illustrated and do not include anatomical sketches, line drawings for surgical guidance, or any other visual depictions of the medical body; representations of the medical body in the Ayurvedic tradition do not appear in the Indian subcontinent until the eighteenth century (Wujastyk 2009). The medical illustrations from Chinese and Western cultures evolved to reflect a number of distinct genres, each with different aims. In some cases, the pictures may have been designed merely to be aesthetically pleasing or humorous, like the images of people representing different humoral types in medieval Europe—a series of four pictures showing the personality of a man whose temperament was controlled by each of the four humors. In addition to providing aesthetically pleasing pictures, however, many illustrations also served a more didactic purpose.

One of the most common genres of medical illustration portrayed the human body to reflect upon the interaction between the microcosm and the macrocosm. In Western art, the "zodiac man" usually displayed a human with the signs of the zodiac placed over the parts of the body with which they were thought to exert an influence (Capricorn on the head, Pisces with the feet, Cancer with the chest, etc.) In these figures, the point is to show the human body as the microcosm and how it relates to the wider universe, the macrocosm. One example from Chinese art, the *Neijing Tu* (*Diagram of the Inner Realm*), found on a stone stele in the Baigunguan Temple in Beijing, displays the body as a macrocosm. The head is shown as a mountainous landscape with rapids descending from it and continuing down the spinal column to the ocean below the abdomen, the torso contains a forest, and the abdominal region has an ox pulling a plough through fields where crops are being sown. Human figures are also arrayed in the picture, such as a white-haired old man in a yoga pose in the head and a pretty girl by a spinning wheel in the upper abdomen. Carefully interpreted as a whole, the *Neijing Tu* reveals certain Taoist medico-alchemical concepts of the body, the relationship between the microcosm and the macrocosm, and the quest to prolong life and attain immortality. Slightly different versions of the *Neijing Tu* exist, but all reflect the same basic concepts (see illustration on p. 12).

Other medical images are designed to offer guidance on treatment. In the West, where bloodletting was a primary therapeutic action, figures of the "bloodletting man" were common, depicting a human body with the major veins marked, sometimes with notations indicating specific locations where one could let blood. Some images did double duty, combining the "zodiac man" and "bloodletting man" figures (see illustration on p. 226). These figures were similar to depictions of the "wound man" (see illustration on p. 194) and "disease man" (see illustration on p. 66), which again showed the human body either with text describing diseases with arrows indicating the parts of the body

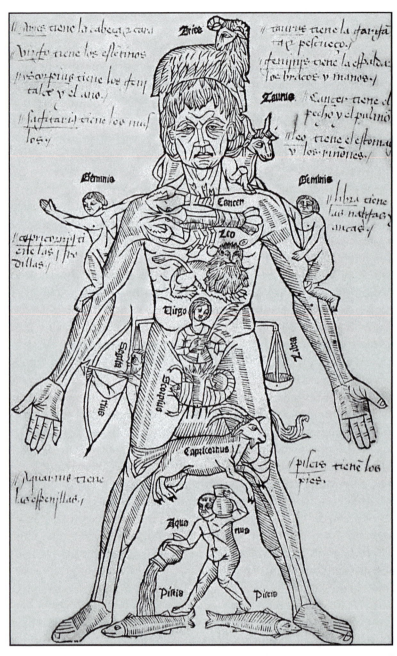

This is a "zodiac man" illustration from a medieval European manuscript. The zodiac man was a typical genre of illustration in medieval manuscripts in which the signs of the zodiac were drawn over the parts of the body they were believed to influence. These charts reflect the prevalent belief in the role of astrological influences on individual health. (National Library of Medicine)

they afflicted, or with images of the kinds of gruesome wounds a body could receive. In China, images of the body were depicted not to indicate bloodletting points, but rather to mark out sites for the application of acupuncture and moxibustion. In many cases, these images were even updated to reflect changes in theory or practice. For example, the famous Tang physician Sun Simiao (581–682 C.E.) was concerned that older illustrations may contain errors and show the wrong points for acupuncture and sought to create newer more accurate drawings to teach practitioners (see illustration on p. 166).

The study of human anatomy developed in different ways in China and the West, but in both cases it was linked to the depiction of anatomical structures in art. Opening dead bodies was seldom practiced in ancient China due to traditional beliefs about the sacredness of the body and taboos about disfiguring bodies for any reasons. During the Song dynasty (960–1279 C.E.), however, some texts recount efforts to dissect dead bodies for the purposes of studying human anatomy. In the first case, from around 1045, the bandit Ou Xifan was executed and, at the command of the local governor, his body was delivered to physicians so that it could be dissected and drawings could be made of the internal structures (some versions of this recount that his body was dissected along with those of some fifty fellow bandits). Later, the physician Yang Jie (1068–1140) produced a volume of anatomical drawings also based upon the dissection of executed criminals who were delivered for this purpose by the local governor. It is significant that in both of these cases, the dissection took place with the express intention of producing illustrated textbooks of human anatomy. Unfortunately, copies of the books that were produced do not exist today and their illustrations are lost. The study of human anatomy did not receive extensive attention in later periods of Chinese history, which no doubt reflects the continued taboos against opening dead bodies, but also the fact that a detailed understanding of human anatomy was not deemed necessary for the proper application of traditional Chinese medicine. Nonetheless, images of internal anatomy continued to circulate in medical texts, perhaps copies of those originally drawn from the dissection of criminals. In these images, internal organs are not depicted as distinct entities, with a recognizable shape or form and were usually intended to depict the *zang* and *fu* organs in relation to specific acupuncture points. As such, they would not have been especially useful for learning sufficient anatomical detail for success in surgery, but they would have helped elicit principles of theoretical importance for physicians interested in knowing the number of orifices in the throat or the position of the liver in relation to important acupuncture points (see illustration on p. 52).

Whereas the practice of human dissection was limited in other ancient cultures it came to be considered a necessary component of a physician's medical training in the medieval European universities. Starting in Bologna shortly after 1300, many universities began to perform public dissections of two or three human bodies (criminal bodies, preferably at least one male and one female) once per year (usually in winter to minimize the effects of putrefaction) for the purposes of teaching human anatomy. The dissection would be held in a church or a temporary lecture hall, hastily built for the occasion, and would take place over the course of about one week, during which time the dissectors would focus on revealing the organs of the three main body cavities (abdomen, thorax, and head). The labor of the procedure itself was divided among three main participants: a senior student, who would read a relevant passage from an anatomical text concerning the structure about to be revealed, a surgeon, who would do the actual cutting, and a professor of medicine (a physician), who would point out the structure and add additional commentary as a means of teaching the material discussed in the text. Pictures of a university dissection scene became common in the later Middle Ages and they serve to emphasize a number of points, including social distinctions between the theoretical learning of the physician and the manual craft practice of the surgeon. These illustrations of physicians studying anatomy thus came to signify their theoretical training, just like the images of the physician holding a urine flask (see illustration on p. 38).

A number of anatomical texts were written that included illustrations of the structures of internal anatomy, the most famous being that by Mondino de' Liuzzi (ca. 1270–1326), the *Anathomia corporis humani* (*Anatomy of the Human Body*). The most common illustrations were the five figure series, pictures of squatting men each of whom depicted a major anatomical structure: artery man, vein man (similar to the blood-letting man figures), nerve man, skeleton man, and muscle man. These illustrations were typically highly schematic and did not necessarily seek to provide an accurate depiction of the body parts (e.g., skeleton man would often have the wrong number of ribs, while muscle man was usually shown with a characteristic donut shaped muscle around the stomach). Other illustrations depicted a body with the major organs on it, usually including the lungs, heart, stomach, liver, kidneys, and intestines. While these illustrations often did more to distinguish the major organs from one another and give rough attention to their shape than the Chinese organ illustrations, they were still highly schematic.

Given the fact that students would have had little opportunity for hands-on examination of the bodies during the dissection lessons, it is unlikely that they learned much anatomical detail during them, so medical students were mostly expected to learn anatomy by reading textbooks. Likewise, the illustrations they could view in these texts would not have conveyed enough detail to offer practical guidance for surgery. However, as with the Chinese illustrations, they were detailed enough to help answer significant theoretical questions of interest to the physician, who did not otherwise need to have an exceedingly detailed knowledge of anatomy for successful practice. In 1543, Andreas Vesalius (1514–1564) published his *De Humani Corporis Fabrica (On the Fabric of the Human Body)*, a lavishly illustrated anatomical textbook, which revolutionized the study of anatomy and anatomical illustration. Vesalius's pictures aimed at providing accurate depictions of the shape of organs and their positions within the body, drawing a sharp contrast in terms of the detail and goals to previous anatomical illustrations from the Middle Ages and those produced in China.

# Glossary

**acupuncture**—the therapeutic practice common in traditional Chinese medicine in which needles are applied at specific sites on the body to redirect the flow of *qi* and restore health.

*ashipu*—the exorcist, or priest, who treated the sick in ancient Mesopotamia with charms, drugs, and magical cures.

*asu*—the physician in ancient Mesopotamia, who treated the sick with charms, drugs, and magical cures.

**Ayurvedic medicine**—*Ayurveda* literally means "knowledge for longevity." This is the medical tradition in India based on the oral traditions passed on by practicing healers from the Vedic period (ca. 1500–500 B.C.E). Ayurvedic medicine emphasizes rational or naturalistic medical knowledge but also incorporates magical healing traditions.

**bloodletting**—the therapeutic practice used in several premodern cultures, but most common in the humoral tradition practiced in Greece, Rome, the Islamic world, and medieval Europe. Small amounts of blood would be let from various parts of the body (typically by cutting open veins, but also through applying leeches) in order to remove unhealthy humors from the body and thus restore a healthy humoral balance.

*chirurgicus*—the surgeon in medieval Europe.

**cupping**—the therapeutic practice in which the doctor would put a piece of burning material into a little metal or glass cup so that when applied to the skin, the flame would be extinguished and create a vacuum, holding the cup to the skin. The suction was believed to help draw internal humors to the site, to help rectify localized humoral imbalances in the body and restore health. The practice of "wet" cupping (as opposed to "dry" cupping) entailed scarifying the skin to cause bleeding before applying the cup, so that harmful excess humors could be drawn out of the body.

*dhatus*—the seven basic structural constituents (tissues and fluids) of the body in Ayurvedic medicine: *rasa* (plasma or chyle), *rakta* (blood), *mamsa* (muscle and flesh), *meda* (fat), *asthi* (bone), *majjan* (marrow and nerve tissue), and *shukra* (semen).

*doshas*—the concept in Ayurvedic medicine of humors or substances in the body required for its proper functioning. They are *vata* (wind or air), *pitta* (bile or fire), and *kapha* (phlegm or water). They are transported through the body through a network of channels or tubes called *srotas*.

**Hippocratic Corpus**—the body of approximately sixty texts written from 450 to 350 B.C.E. and ascribed to Hippocrates. These texts are often mutually contradictory and reflect different dialects, indicating that they were not likely written by a single individual. It is not clear which, if any, of these texts may have been written by the real Hippocrates.

**humoralism**—the theoretical system originating in Greek medicine that envisions the body as a being composed of four humors: blood, phlegm, black bile (melancholy), and yellow bile (choler). According to humoral theory, disease arises when the humors are out of balance in the body. Humoralism was central to the medical practices in Greece, Rome, the Islamic world, and the medieval West.

*iatros* **(pl.** *iatroi***)**—the physician in ancient Greece.

*malas*—the main waste products of the body produced as a result of digestion in Ayurvedic medicine: feces, urine, and sweat. The maintenance of health requires that these be effectively eliminated from the body.

**moxibustion**—the therapeutic practice common in traditional Chinese medicine in which mugwort tinder (moxa) is used to cause a burn on specific points of the body, typically to help redirect the flow of *qi* in the body and restore health.

**naturalistic medicine**—medical beliefs that explain health and disease as a rational and natural process in which gods and supernatural beings are not involved.

*physicus*—the university trained physician in medieval Europe, as distinguished from the *medicus*, or doctor who may or may not have earned a university degree.

*qi*—the concept in Traditional Chinese medicine translated as "vapor," "breath," or "energy" and recognized as the vital principle that flows through meridians or pathways in the body and is essential for promoting growth and the healthy operation of the body.

*swnw*—the physician in ancient Egypt.

**systematic correspondence**—the concept present in many pre-modern medical theories by which the actions of the universe (macrocosm) are connected to and exert and influence on the functioning of the human body (microcosm).

*vaidyas*—physicians in Ayurvedic medicine.

*wu xing*—the concept in traditional Chinese medicine of the "five phases" or "five elements" (wood, fire, earth, metal, and water), which compose the universe and the body.

# Suggestions for Further Reading

## Selected Primary Sources in English Translation

Albucasis. *Albucasis on Surgery and Instruments: A Definitive Edition of the Arabic Text with English Translation and Commentary.* Translated by M.S. Spink and G.L. Lewis. London: The Wellcome Institute of the History of Medicine, 1973.

Bhishagratna, Kaviraj Kunjalal. *An English Translation of the Sushruta Samhita Based on Original Sanskrit Text with a Full and Comprehensive Introduction, Additional Texts, Different Readings, Notes, Comparative Views, Index, Glossary and Plates.* 3 vols. Calcutta: J.N. Bose, 1907–1916.

Breasted, James Henry. *The Edwin Smith Surgical Papyrus.* Vol. 1. Chicago: University of Chicago Press, 1930.

Bryan, Cyril P. *Ancient Egyptian Medicine: The Papyrus Ebers.* Chicago: Ares Publishers Inc., 1974.

Celsus. *De Medicina.* 3 vols. Translated by Walter George Spencer. Loeb Classical Library. Cambridge, MA: Harvard University Press, 1935–1938.

Chuncai, Zhou, and Han Yazhou. *The Illustrated Yellow Emperor's Canon of Medicine.* Beijing: Dolphin Books, 1997.

Galen. *Method of Medicine.* 3 vols. Translated by Ian Johnston and G.H.R. Horsley. Loeb Classical Library. Cambridge, MA: Harvard University Press, 2011.

Galen. *On the Natural Faculties.* Translated by A.W. Brock. Loeb Classical Library. Cambridge, MA: Harvard University Press, 1979.

Garrison, Daniel, ed. *A Cultural History of the Human Body.* Vol. 1, *In Antiquity (1000 BC–500 AD).* Oxford: Berg Publishers, 2010.

Gunther, Robert T. *The Greek Herbal of Dioscorides.* New York: Hafner Publishing Co., 1959.

*Hippocrates.* 9 vols. Translated by W.H.S. Jones, E. T. Withington, Paul Potter, and Wesley D. Smith. Loeb Classical Library. Cambridge, MA: Harvard University Press, 1923–2010.

Horrox, Rosemary. *The Black Death.* Manchester: Manchester University Press, 1994.

Lemay, Helen Rodnite. *Women's Secrets: A Translation of Pseudo-Albertus Magnus's* De Secretis Mulierum *with Commentaries.* Albany: State University of New York Press, 1992.

Ni, Maoshing. *The Yellow Emperor's Classic of Medicine: A New Translation of the* Neijing Suwen *with Commentary.* London: Shambhala, 1995.

Sharma, Priya Vrat. *Susruta-Samhita with English Translation of Text and Dalhana's Commentary along with Critical Notes.* 3 vols. Varanasi, India: Chaukhambha Visvabharati, 1999–2001.

Sharma, Ram Karan, and Vaidya Bhagwan Dash. *Agnivesa's* Caraka Samhita: *Text with English Translation & Critical Exposition.* 6 vols. Varanasi, India: Chowkhamba Sanskrit Series Office, 1976–2001.

Temkin, Owsei. *Soranus' Gynecology.* Baltimore, MD: Johns Hopkins University Press, 1956.

Teodorico Borgognoni. *The Surgery of Theodoric, ca. A.D. 1267.* Vol. 1. Translated by Eldridge Campbell and James Colton. New York: Appleton-Century-Crofts, Inc., 1955.

Veith, Ilza. *Huang Ti Nei Ching Su Wên: The Yellow Emperor's Classic of Internal Medicine,* New ed. Berkeley: University of California Press, 1972.

Wujastyk, Dominik. *The Roots of Ayurveda: Selections from Sanskrit Medical Writings.* New York: Penguin Books, 2003.

## Selected Modern Works

Auboyer, Jeannine. *Daily Life in Ancient India, from Approximately 200 B.C. to 700 A.D.* New York: Macmillan, 1965.

Biggs, Robert D. "Medicine and Public Health in Ancient Mesopotamia." *Journal of Assyrian Academic Studies* 19 (2005): 1–19.

Byrne, Joseph P. *Daily Life during the Black Death.* Westport, CT: Greenwood Press, 2006.

Cameron, M. L. *Anglo-Saxon Medicine.* Cambridge, MA: Cambridge University Press, 1993.

Conrad, Lawrence I., Michael Neve, Vivian Nutton, Roy Porter, and Andrew Wear, eds. *The Western Medical Tradition: 800 BC to AD 1800.* Cambridge, MA: Cambridge University Press, 1995.

Conrad, Lawrence I., and Dominik Wujastyk, eds. *Contagion: Perspectives from Pre-Modern Societies.* Aldershot: Ashgate, 2000.

Cruse, Audrey. *Roman Medicine.* Stroud, Gloucestershire: Tempus, 2004.

Demaitre, Luke. *Leprosy in Premodern Medicine: A Malady of the Whole Body.* Baltimore, MD: Johns Hopkins University Press, 2007.

Desai, Prakash N. *Health and Medicine in the Hindu Tradition: Continuity and Cohesion.* New York: Crossroad Publishing Company, 1989.

Dols, Michael W. *The Black Death in the Middle East.* Princeton, NJ: Princeton University Press, 1977.

Dols, Michael W. *Majnun: The Madman in Medieval Islamic Society.* Edited by Diana E. Immisch. Oxford: Clarendon Press, 1992.

Furth, Charlotte. *A Flourishing Yin: Gender in China's Medical History, 960–1665.* Berkeley: University of California Press, 1999.

Gernet, Jacques. *Daily Life in China on the Eve of the Mongol Invasion 1250–1276.* Translated by H.M. Wright. Stanford, CA: Stanford University Press, 1962.

Goldschmidt, Asaf. *The Evolution of Chinese Medicine: Song Dynasty, 960–1200.* New York: Routledge, 2009.

Green, Monica H. *Making Women's Medicine Masculine: The Rise of Male Authority in Pre-Modern Gynaecology.* Oxford: Oxford University Press, 2008.

Hanawalt, Barbara A. *Growing Up in Medieval London: The Experience of Childhood in History.* Oxford: Oxford University Press, 1993.

Hanawalt, Barbara A. *The Ties That Bound: Peasant Families in Medieval England.* Oxford: Oxford University Press, 1986.

Hoizey, Dominique, and Marie-Joseph. *A History of Chinese Medicine.* Translated by Paul Bailey. Edinburgh: Edinburgh University Press, 1993.

Hopkins, Donald R. *The Greatest Killer: Smallpox in History.* Chicago: University of Chicago Press, 1983.

Jolly, Julius. *Indian Medicine.* Translated by C.G. Kashikar. New Delhi: Munshiram Manoharlal, 1994.

Kalof, Linda, ed. *A Cultural History of the Human Body.* Vol. 2, *In the Medieval Age (1000–1400).* Oxford: Berg Publishers, 2010.

Kuriyama, Shigehisa. *The Expressiveness of the Body and the Divergence of Greek and Chinese Medicine.* New York: Zone Books, 1999.

Leung, Angela Ki Che. *Leprosy in China: A History.* New York: Columbia University Press, 2008.

Majno, Guido. *The Healing Hand: Man and Wound in the Ancient World.* Cambridge, MA: Harvard University Press, 1975.

Mazars, Guy. *A Concise Introduction to Indian Medicine.* Delhi: Motilal Banarsidass Publishers, 2006.

McNeill, William H. *Plagues and Peoples.* Garden City, NY: Anchor Press, 1976.

McVaugh, Michael R. *Medicine before the Plague: Practitioners and Their Patients in the Crown of Aragon, 1285–1345.* Cambridge, MA: Cambridge University Press, 1993.

McVaugh, Michael R. *The Rational Surgery of the Middle Ages.* Florence: Sismel—Edizioni del Galluzzo, 2006.

Ng, Vivian W. *Madness in Late Imperial China: From Illness to Deviance.* Norman: University of Oklahoma Press, 1990.

Nunn, John F. *Ancient Egyptian Medicine.* Norman: University of Oklahoma Press, 1996.

Nutton, Vivian. *Ancient Medicine.* New York: Routledge, 2004.

Park, Katharine. "Medicine and Society in Medieval Europe, 500–1500." In *Medicine in Society: Historical Essays*, edited by Andrew Wear, 59–90. Cambridge, MA: Cambridge University Press, 1992.

Park, Katharine. *Secrets of Women: Gender, Generation, and the Origins of Human Dissection*. New York: Zone, 2010.

Pormann, Peter E., and Emilie Savage-Smith. *Medieval Islamic Medicine*. Washington, DC: Georgetown University Press, 2007.

Rawcliffe, Carole. *Leprosy in Medieval England*. Rochester: Boydell Press, 2006.

Riddle, John M. *Contraception and Abortion from the Ancient World to the Renaissance*. Cambridge, MA: Harvard University Press, 1992.

Robson, Eleanor. "Mesopotamian Medicine & Religion: Current Debates, New Perspectives." *Religion Compass* 2, no. 4 (2008): 455–83.

Salazar, Christine F. *The Treatment of War Wounds in Graeco-Roman Antiquity*. Leiden: Brill, 2000.

Scarborough, John. *Roman Medicine*. Ithaca, NY: Cornell University Press, 1969.

Sharma, Priya Vrat. *Indian Medicine in the Classical Age*. Varanasi, India: Chowkhamba Sanskrit Series Office, 1972.

Siraisi, Nancy G. *Medieval and Early Renaissance Medicine: An Introduction to Knowledge and Practice*. Chicago: University of Chicago Press, 1990.

Stol, M. *Epilepsy in Babylonia*. Groningen: Styx, 1993.

Strickmann, Michel. *Chinese Magical Medicine*. Stanford, CA: Stanford University Press, 2002.

Thompson, R. Campbell. *Assyrian Medical Texts*. London: John Bale Sons & Danielsson, Ltd., 1924.

Unschuld, Paul U. *Medicine in China: A History of Ideas*. Berkeley: University of California Press, 1985.

Ware, James R. *Alchemy, Medicine, Religion in the China of A.D. 320: The Nei P'ien of Ko Hung (Pao-p'u tzu)*. Cambridge, MA: MIT Press, 1966.

White, David Gordon. *The Alchemical Body: Siddha Traditions in Medieval India*. Chicago: University of Chicago Press, 1996.

Zhenguo, Wang, Chen Ping, and Xie Peiping. *History and Development of Traditional Chinese Medicine*. Vol. 1. Beijing: Science Press, 1999.

Ziegler, Philip. *Black Death*. New York: John Day Co., 1969.

Zysk, Kenneth G. *Asceticism and Healing in Ancient India: Medicine in the Buddhist Monastery*. 2nd ed. Delhi: Motilal Banarsidass, 1998.

# Bibliography

Amulree, Lord. "Hygienic Conditions in Ancient Rome and Modern London." *Medical History* 17 (1973): 244–55.

Archer, Christon I., John R. Ferris, Holger H. Herwig, and Timothy H. E. Travers. *World History of Warfare*. Lincoln: University of Nebraska Press, 2002.

Bhishagratna, Kaviraj Kunjalal. *An English Translation of the Sushruta Samhita Based on Original Sanskrit Text*. Vol. 1, *Sutrasthanam*. Calcutta: No. 10, Kashi Ghose's Lane, 1907.

Bhishagratna, Kaviraj Kunjalal. *An English Translation of the Sushruta Samhita with a Full and Comprehensive Introduction, Additional Texts, Different Readings, Notes, Comparative Views, Index, Glossary and Plates*. Vol. 2, *Nidana-Sthana, S'Arira-Sthana, Chikitsita-Sthana and Kalapa-Sthana*. Calcutta: No. 10, Kashi Ghose's Lane, 1911.

Biggs, Robert D. "Medicine and Public Health in Ancient Mesopotamia." *Journal of Assyrian Academic Studies* 19, no. 1 (2005): 1–19.

Bloomfield, M. *Hymns of the Atharva Veda*. Whitefish, MT: Kessinger Publishing, 2004.

Boer, Charles. *Marsilio Ficino's Book of Life*. Woodstock, CT: Spring Publications, 1980.

Boylston, Anthea. "Evidence for Weapon-Related Trauma in British Archaeological Samples." In *Human Osteology in Archaeology and Forensic Science*, edited by M. Cox and S. Mays, 357–80. London: Greenwich Medical Media, 2000.

Breasted, James Henry. *The Edwin Smith Surgical Papyrus*. Vol. 1. Chicago: University of Chicago Press, 1930.

Bryan, Cyril P. *Ancient Egyptian Medicine: The Papyrus Ebers.* Chicago: Ares Publishers Inc., 1974.

Caciola, Nancy. *Discerning Spirits: Divine and Demonic Possession in the Middle Ages.* Ithaca, NY: Cornell University Press, 2003.

Campbell, Eldridge, and James Colton, trans. *The Surgery of Theodoric, ca. A.D. 1267.* Vol. 1. New York: Appleton-Century-Crofts, Inc., 1955.

Carmichael, Ann G. *Plague and the Poor in Renaissance Florence.* Cambridge, MA: Cambridge University Press, 1986.

Chadwick, J., and W.N. Mann, trans. *Hippocratic Writings,* edited by G.E.R. Lloyd. New York: Penguin Books, 1950.

Chiu, Martha Li. "Insanity in Imperial China: A Legal Case Study." In *Normal and Abnormal Behavior in Chinese Culture*, edited by Arthur Kleinman and Tsung-Yi Lin, 75–94. Dordrecht: D. Reidel Publishing Co., 1981.

Cholmeley, H.P. *John of Gaddesden and the Rosa Medicinae.* Oxford: Clarendon Press, 1912.

Cruse, Audrey. *Roman Medicine.* Stroud, Gloucestershire: Tempus Publishing, 2004.

Demaitre, Luke E. *Doctor Bernard de Gordon: Professor and Practitioner.* Toronto: Pontifical Institute of Mediaeval Studies, 1980.

Demaitre, Luke. "The Care and Extension of Old Age in Medieval Medicine." In *Aging and the Aged in Medieval Europe*, edited by Michael M. Sheehan, 3–22. Toronto: Pontifical Institute of Mediaeval Studies, 1990.

Demaitre, Luke. "The Idea of Childhood and Child Care in Medical Writings of the Middle Ages." *Journal of Psychohistory* 4 (1977): 461–90.

Demaitre, Luke. *Leprosy in Premodern Medicine: A Malady of the Whole Body.* Baltimore, MD: Johns Hopkins University Press, 2007.

Dols, Michael W. *The Black Death in the Middle East.* Princeton, NJ: Princeton University Press, 1977.

Dols, Michael W. *Majnun: The Madman in Medieval Islamic Society*, edited by Diana E. Immisch. Oxford: Clarendon Press, 1992.

Edelstein, Emma J., and Ludwig Edelstein. *Asclepius: Collection and Interpretation of the Testimonies.* Vols. 1 and 2. Baltimore, MD: Johns Hopkins University Press, 1998.

Edelstein, Ludwig. *Ancient Medicine: Selected Papers of Ludwig Edelstein,* edited by Owsei Temkin and C. Lilian Temkin. Baltimore, MD: Johns Hopkins University Press, 1967.

Fagles, Robert, trans. Homer, *The Iliad.* New York: Penguin Books, 1990.

Fagles, Robert, trans. Homer, *The Odyssey.* New York: Penguin Books, 1996.

Finucane, Ronald C. *Miracles and Pilgrims: Popular Beliefs in Medieval England.* London: J.M. Dent & Sons, Ltd., 1977.

Furth, Charlotte. *A Flourishing Yin: Gender in China's Medical History, 960–1665.* Berkeley: University of California Press, 1999.

Ghalioungui, Paul. *Magic and Medical Science in Ancient Egypt.* New York: Barnes & Noble, Inc., 1963.

Gies, Joseph, and Frances Gies. *Life in a Medieval City.* London: The Folio Society, 2002.

Green, Monica H. *Making Women's Medicine Masculine: The Rise of Male Authority in Pre-Modern Gynaecology.* Oxford: Oxford University Press, 2008.

Grene, David, trans. Herodotus. *The History.* Chicago: University of Chicago Press, 1987.

Guihua, Xie. "Han Bamboo and Wooden Medical Records Discovered in Military Sites from the North-Western Frontier Regions." In *Medieval Chinese Medicine: The Dunhuang Medical Manuscripts,* edited by Vivienne Lo and Christopher Cullen, 78–106. London: Routledge, 2005.

Gunther, Robert T. *The Greek Herbal of Dioscorides.* New York: Hafner Publishing Co., 1959.

Hanawalt, Barbara A. *Growing Up in Medieval London: The Experience of Childhood in History.* Oxford: Oxford University Press, 1993.

Hanawalt, Barbara A. *The Ties That Bound: Peasant Families in Medieval England.* Oxford: Oxford University Press, 1986.

Hanson, Ann Ellis. "Diseases of Women 1." *Signs* 1 (1975): 567–584.

Hopkins, Donald R. *The Greatest Killer: Smallpox in History.* Chicago: University of Chicago Press, 1983.

Horrox, Rosemary. *The Black Death.* Manchester: Manchester University Press, 1994.

Jones, Frederic Wood. "Some lessons from ancient fractures." *British Medical Journal* 2 (August 22, 1908): 455–458.

Jones, Peter Murray. "John of Arderne and the Mediterranean Tradition of Scholastic Surgery." In *Practical Medicine from Salerno to the Black Death,* edited by Luis García-Ballester, Roger French, Jon Arrizabalaga, and Andrew Cunningham, 289–321. Cambridge, MA: Cambridge University Press, 1994.

Jones, W.H.S., trans. Hippocrates, "Airs, Waters, Places" and "Epidemics I and III." In *Hippocrates,* 1:65–137 and 139–287. Cambridge, MA: Harvard University Press, 1984.

Jones, W.H.S., trans. Pliny, *Natural History.* Vol. 7. Cambridge, MA: Harvard University Press, 1956.

Jones, W.H.S., trans. Pliny, *Natural History.* Vol. 8. Cambridge, MA: Harvard University Press, 1963.

Jones, W.H.S., trans. Hippocrates, "On the Sacred Disease." In *Hippocrates,* 2:129–83. Cambridge, MA: Harvard University Press, 1923.

Kutumbiah, P. *Ancient Indian Medicine.* Chennai, India: Orient Longman, 1962.

Lambert, W.G. "The Gula Hymn of Bulluùsa-rabi." *Orientalia,* n. s. 36 (1967): 105-121.

Lemay, Helen Rodnite. *Women's Secrets: A Translation of Pseudo-Albertus Magnus's De Secretis Mulierum with Commentaries.* Albany: State University of New York Press, 1992.

Leung, Angela Ki Che. *Leprosy in China: A History.* New York: Columbia University Press, 2008.

Levey, Martin. *The Medical Formulary or Aqrabadhin of Al-Kindi*. Madison: University of Wisconsin Press, 1966.

Lonie, I. M., trans. *The Hippocratic Treatises on Generation, on the Nature of the Child, Diseases IV: A Commentary*. Berlin: Walter de Gruyter, 1981.

Mair, Victor H., trans. "The Biography of Hua-t'o from the *History of the Three Kingdoms*." In *The Columbia Anthology of Traditional Chinese Literature*, edited by Victor H. Mair, 688–96. New York: Columbia University Press, 1994.

Majno, Guido. *The Healing Hand: Man and Wound in the Ancient World*. Cambridge, MA: Harvard University Press, 1975.

McLeod, Katrina C. D., and Robin D. S. Yates, "Forms of Ch'in Law: An Annotated Translation of the Feng-chen shih." *Harvard Journal of Asiatic Studies* 41 (1981): 111–63.

McVaugh, Michael R. *Arnaldi de Villanova Opera Medica Omnia*. Vol. 2, *Aphorismi de Gradibus*. Granada and Barcelona: Seminarium Historiae Medicae Granatensis, 1975.

McVaugh, Michael R. "Cataracts and Hernias: Aspects of Surgical Practice in the Fourteenth Century." *Medical History* 45 (2001): 319–40.

McVaugh, Michael R. "Incantations in Late Medieval Surgery." In *Ratio et Superstitio: Essays in Honor of Graziella Frederici Vescovini*, edited by Giancarlo Marchetti, Orsola Rignani and Valeria Sorge, 319–46. Leuvene-la-Neuve, Belgium: Fédération Internationale des Instituts d'Etudes Médiévale, 2003.

McVaugh, Michael R. *The Rational Surgery of the Middle Ages*. Florence: Sismel—Edizioni del Galluzzo, 2006.

McWilliam, G. H., trans. Giovanni Boccaccio, *The Decameron*. New York: Penguin Books, 1995.

Meek, Theophile J., trans. "The Code of Hammurabi." In *Ancient Near Eastern Texts Relating to the Old Testament*, 3rd ed. with Supplement, edited by James B. Pritchard, 163–80. Princeton, NJ: Princeton University Press, 1969.

Ng, Vivian W. *Madness in Late Imperial China: From Illness to Deviance*. Norman: University of Oklahoma Press, 1990.

Ni, Maoshing. *The Yellow Emperor's Classic of Medicine: A New Translation of the Neijing Suwen with Commentary*. Boston, MA: Shambhala, 1995.

Nriagu, Jerome O. "Occupational Exposure to Lead in Ancient Times." *Science of the Total Environment* 31 (1983): 105–16.

Nunn, John F. *Ancient Egyptian Medicine*. Norman: University of Oklahoma Press, 1996.

Oppenheim, A. Leo. "The Mother of Nabodinus." In *Ancient Near Eastern Texts Relating to the Old Testament*, 3rd edition with Supplement, edited by James B. Pritchard, 560–62. Princeton, NJ: Princeton University Press, 1969.

Park, Katharine. "Birth and Death." In *A Cultural History of the Human Body in the Medieval Age*, edited by Linda Kalof, 17–38. Oxford: Berg Publishers, 2010.

Park, Katharine. "Medicine and Society in Medieval Europe, 500–1500." In *Medicine in Society: Historical Essays*, edited by Andrew Wear, 59–90. Cambridge, MA: Cambridge University Press, 1992.

Pormann, Peter E., and Emilie Savage-Smith. *Medieval Islamic Medicine.* Washington, DC: Georgetown University Press, 2007.

Potter, Paul, trans. "On Haemorrhoids." In *Hippocrates,* 8:377–89. Cambridge, MA: Harvard University Press, 1995.

Riddle, John M. *Contraception and Abortion from the Ancient World to the Renaissance.* Cambridge, MA: Harvard University Press, 1992.

Robbins, G., V.M. Tripathy, V.N. Misra, R.K. Mohanty, V. S. Shinde, et al. "Ancient Skeletal Evidence for Leprosy in India (2000 B.C.)," *PLoS ONE* 4, no. 5 (2009): e5669. Doi: 10.1371/journal.pone.0005669.

Russell, John Malcolm. "Bulls for the Palace and Order in the Empire: The Sculptural Program of Sennacherib's Court VI at Nineveh." *The Art Bulletin* 69 (1987): 520–539.

Salazar, Christine F. *The Treatment of War Wounds in Graeco-Roman Antiquity.* Leiden: Brill, 2000.

Savage-Smith, Emilie. "The Practice of Surgery in Islamic Lands: Myth and Reality," *Social History of Medicine* 13 (2000): 307–21.

Schipper, Kristofer. *The Taoist Body.* Translated by Karen C. Duval. Berkeley: University of California Press, 1993.

Scurlock, J.A. "Baby-Snatching Demons, Restless Souls and the Dangers of Childbirth: Medico-Magical Means of Dealing with Some of the Perils of Motherhood in Ancient Mesopotamia." *Incognita* 2 (1991): 135–183.

Seward, Desmond. *The Hundred Years War: The English in France, 1337–1453.* New York: Atheneum, 1978.

Shahar, Meir. *Crazy Ji: Chinese Religion and Popular Literature.* Cambridge, Mass.: Harvard University Press, 1998.

Sharma, Priya Vrat. *Susruta-Samhita with English Translation of Text and Dalhana's Commentary Alongwith Critical Notes.* Vol. 1, *Sutrasthana.* Varanasi, India: Chaukhambha Visvabharati, 1999.

Sharma, Ram Karan, and Vaidya Bhagwan Dash. *Agnivesa's* Caraka Samhita*: Text with English Translation & Critical Exposition.* Varanasi, India: Chowkhamba Sanskrit Series Office, 1976.

Sigerist, Henry E. *A History of Medicine.* Vol. 1, *Primitive and Archaic Medicine.* Oxford: Oxford University Press, 1951.

Spencer, W. G., trans. Celsus, *De Medicina.* Vol. 2. Cambridge, MA: Harvard University Press, 1953.

Spencer, W.G., trans. Celsus, *De Medicina.* Vol. 3. Cambridge, MA: Harvard University Press, 1961.

Spink, M.S., and G.L. Lewis. *Albucasis On Surgery and Instruments: A Definitive Edition of the Arabic Text with English Translation and Commentary.* London: Wellcome Institute of the History of Medicine, 1973.

Stol, M. *Epilepsy in Babylonia.* Groningen: Styx, 1993.

Temkin, Owsei. *Soranus' Gynecology.* Baltimore, MD: Johns Hopkins University Press, 1956.

Thompson, R. Campbell. *Assyrian Medical Texts.* London: John Bale Sons & Danielsson, Ltd., 1924.

Veith, Ilza. *Huang Ti Nei Ching Su Wên: The Yellow Emperor's Classic of Internal Medicine.* New Edition. Berkeley: University of California Press, 1972.

Veith, Ilza. "The Supernatural in Far Eastern Concepts of Mental Disease." *Bulletin of the History of Medicine* 37 (1963): 139–158.

Ware, James R. *Alchemy, Medicine, Religion in the China of A.D. 320: The Nei P'ien of Ko Hung (Pao-p'u tzu).* Cambridge, MA: MIT Press, 1966.

Wilson, John A. "Egyptian Rituals and Incantations." In *Ancient Near Eastern Texts Relating to the Old Testament,* 3rd ed. with Supplement, edited by James B. Pritchard, 325–31. Princeton, NJ: Princeton University Press, 1969.

Withington, E. T., trans. Hippocrates, "On Joints." In *Hippocrates,* 3:201–397. Cambridge, MA: Harvard University Press, 1944a.

Withington, E. T., trans. Hippocrates, "On Wounds in the Head." In *Hippocrates,* 3:1–51. Cambridge, MA: Harvard University Press, 1944b.

Wright, David, trans. Geoffrey Chaucer, *The Canterbury Tales: A Verse Translation with an Introduction and Notes.* Oxford: Oxford University Press, 1985.

Wright, H. M., trans. Jacques Gernet, *Daily Life in China on the Eve of the Mongol Invasion 1250–1276.* Stanford: Stanford University Press, 1962.

Wujastyk, Dominik. "Interpreting the Image of the Human Body in Pre-Modern India." *International Journal of Hindu Studies* 13, no. 2 (2009): 189–228.

Wujastyk, Dominik. *The Roots of Ayurveda: Selections from Sanskrit Medical Writings.* New York: Penguin Books, 2003.

Zhenguo, Wang, Chen Ping, and Xie Peiping. *History and Development of Traditional Chinese Medicine.* Vol. 1. Beijing: Science Press, 1999.

Zysk, Kenneth G. *Asceticism and Healing in Ancient India: Medicine in the Buddhist monastery.* 2nd ed. Delhi: Motilal Banarsidass, 1998.

# Index

Titles of written works are listed under the author's name, when known.

tion of dead fetus, 72; in Greece and Rome, 61–62; in Islamic medicine, 65–67; in medieval Europe, 67–68; menstruation, 61, 62, 64; in Mesopotamia and Egypt, 59–61, 68–71; pregnancy and pregnant women, 24, 44, 47, 63, 68, 69, 71, 74–75, 77–80, 91, 107, 218; in traditional Chinese medicine, 63–64. *See also* Caesarean section; Fertility; Midwifery; Sterility

Haly Abbas. *See* Majusi
Hansen's Disease. *See* Leprosy
Heart, 21, 10, 13–14, 161, 173, 201; in Chinese medicine, 15, 51, 167; seat of intelligence and emotions, 3, 160, 163, 167, 208; source of *metu*, 4; *zang* organ, 15
Henri de Mondeville, 156, 158
Herodotus, 45–46, 86, 178, 208–9
Herophilus, 209–10
Hippocrates of Cos, 5, 22. *See also* Hippocratic Corpus
Hippocratic Corpus, 5, 6, 8, 22–23; *Airs, Waters, Places*, 103–4, 121, 162; *Aphorisms*, 24; *Diseases of Women*, 61; *Epidemics I*, 3; *Oath*, 23, 72, 141; *On Diseases II*, 141–42; *On Generation*, 61; *On the Nature of Man*, 6, 143; *On the Nature of the Child*, 72; *On the Sacred Disease*, 49–50, 161–62; *On Wounds of the Head*, 197
Home design, 122–23, 126–27, 130–32
Homer: *Iliad*, 48
Hospitals, 107, 214, 215, 216–18; education, 35; for insane, 170–71, 172; *leprosaria*, 119, 218; military hospitals, 201–2

*Huangdi Neijing* (*The Yellow Emperor's Classic of Internal Medicine*), 12–13, 29–30, 31, 51, 52–53, 63, 82, 91, 104, 121–22, 151–52, 167–68
Huangfu Mi: *Zhenjiu Jiayijing* (*The ABC of Acupuncture and Moxibustion*), 31, 152
Hua Tuo, 149, 222
Humoralism, 5–6, 82, 143; drug therapy, 190–91; mental state, 162, 172, 225; *See also* Disease, theories of, humoral
Hunayn ibn Ishaq (known as Johannitius in the Latin West), 33; *Isagoge*, 9, 36, 39

*Iatros* (pl. *iatroi*), 23–24, 50, 141
Ibn al-Baytar, 187–89
Ibn Sina (known as Avicenna in the Latin West), 34, 35
Ibn Wahshiyah, 189
Infanticide, 78, 92–93, 96, 218
Insanity. *See* Mental illness
Instruments, surgical, 34, 139, 144, 145, 146, 154, 198
Irrigation. *See* Water supply
Islam: Prophetic medicine, 54–55, 111, 169

Johannitius. *See* Hunayn ibn Ishaq
John of Arderne, 155

Kahun papyrus, 20, 60

Lead poisoning, 129–30
Leprosy, 114–19; in China, 116–18; Hansen's Disease, 114–15; in India, 115–16; *leprosaria*, 119; in medieval Europe, 118–19; responses to, 118–19
Lovesickness, 173–74

Macrocosm, 7, 9, 13, 110–11, 225
Madness. *See* Mental illness

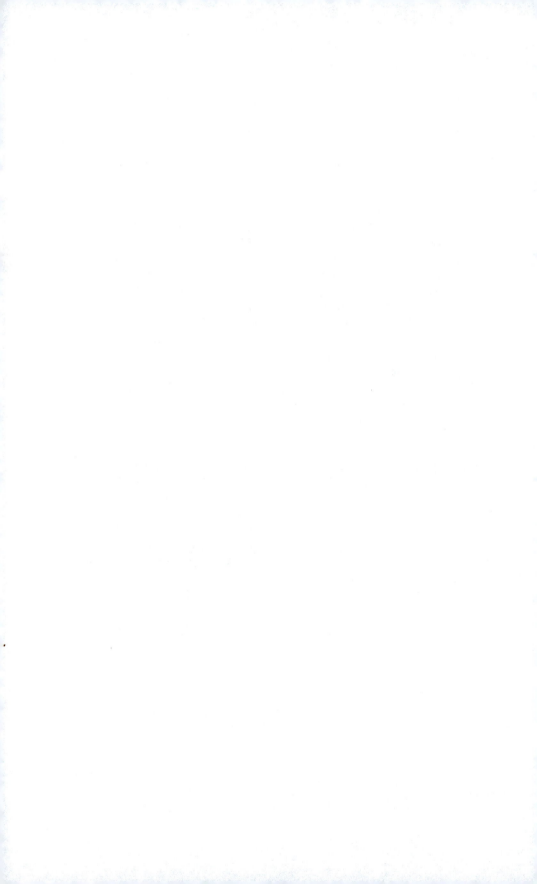

**About the Author**

WILLIAM H. YORK is an assistant professor of interdisciplinary studies in the University Honors Program at Portland State University in Portland, Oregon.